Understanding

COPD
Chronic Obstructive Pulmonary Disease

Dr Daniel K.C. Lee

Published by Family Doctor Publications Limited
in association with the British Medical Association

© Family Doctor Publications 2008

Family Doctor Publications, PO Box 4664, Poole, Dorset BH15 1NN

ISBN-13: 978 1 903474 60 0
ISBN-10: 1 903474 60 4

Contents

About the author

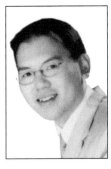

Dr Daniel K.C. Lee, MB, BCh, MRCP, MD, is Associate Professor and Consultant Physician in Respiratory Medicine and General (Internal) Medicine with a prolific publication record of more than 200 publications in peer-reviewed medical journals, having been a graduate in Cardiff, a researcher in Dundee and a trainee in Cambridge.

Introduction

Background to COPD

Chronic obstructive pulmonary disease or COPD affects the lives of people from various communities and different nations. More and more people are being diagnosed with the condition. COPD is very disabling and many people find it hard to cope with the restrictions that it brings.

People with COPD can suffer greatly and many do so in silence. They often wrongly feel that it is their fault that they have developed COPD in the first place and that nothing can be done about it now. Although smoking is the major cause of COPD, it is not the only cause. Being given a diagnosis of COPD is not the same as being handed a death sentence.

COPD imposes limitations on activities of daily living through the symptoms that it causes. It affects the lives of sufferers, carers and the entire community, and also places a significant burden on the health service.

Living with COPD does not have to be a daily struggle. There are medications available that will help to improve symptoms. Practical support is also at hand from various sources ranging from education about COPD to advice on coping with COPD.

This book tries to provide you with a better understanding of COPD. It will give you some insight into the management of the condition. It will also provide you with information on the support network that is available. Living with COPD is no doubt difficult. Understanding it will hopefully make the journey easier.

Case histories
John – mild COPD

John is 50 years old and enjoys playing golf. He has always been a fit and healthy individual. John does not suffer from any medical condition and he does not take any regular medication.

John, however, smokes about 20 cigarettes a day. He has been smoking since he was 20 years old. He attributes his smoking to the stress that he encountered at work. It helps him cope better with the daily strain that he feels.

John took early retirement to spend more time at home with his wife. He started to notice that he got breathless more easily when playing at the golf course. He could no longer walk as far as he used to without first stopping to catch his breath, and also found that he would tire more easily.

Climbing stairs was never a difficulty for him but lately he has been getting breathless when he reaches the top of the stairs. This was obviously worrying him because he could not understand why he should feel this way. After all, he had no health problems that he was aware of.

John's wife also started to notice how he has gradually slowed down and is helping her less with chores at home. This is because he gets tired more easily and is more breathless than usual. He felt that, if he rested more and did less work at home, his condition would improve. It never did. Finally, John decided to see his doctor.

The doctor found that John was mildly wheezy when listening to his chest. John himself had not noticed this wheezing before. A breathing test was performed, which showed evidence of airway narrowing in the lungs. A diagnosis of COPD was made and John was given an inhaler to take whenever he felt breathless.

John is now back playing golf. He is less tired or breathless and is able to do more than before. He finds the inhaler useful and uses it when he gets out of breath. He has also given up smoking. John has mild COPD that is simply controlled with a rescue inhaler.

Comments on case study

It is crucial that John does not start smoking again. Tobacco smoke will irritate the airways in the lungs and cause narrowing, which then leads to breathlessness and wheezing. The inhaler opens up the airways to help with breathing.

If John were to continue smoking, not only would he damage his lungs further, but the tobacco smoke would also fight against the effects of the inhaler. This is because, on the one hand, by taking the inhaler John is keeping his airways opened, but, on the other, by smoking John will cause the airways to narrow.

It is important that you see your doctor should you find that you become easily tired or breathless for no particular reason. This is especially relevant if you are a current smoker or have been a smoker in the past.

The onset of COPD is usually a gradual process and for this reason COPD is sometimes known as 'the silent disease'. You do not necessarily know that your lungs have been damaged by tobacco smoke or that there is airway narrowing in your lungs.

John was not aware that he was wheezing until his doctor examined him. Often people get so used to their limitations and adjust so well to them that they do not realise the gradual deterioration that takes place over time.

Mary – moderate COPD

Mary, a 60-year-old widow and great-grandmother, has been coughing for many years. She says that she feels like she has been coughing all her life but her symptoms really began about 10 years ago. She would cough most mornings and bring up clear thick phlegm. She never took any notice of it at first and accepted that this was simply a smoker's cough.

Mary has been a heavy smoker since she was 12 years old, smoking 20 to 40 cigarettes a day. She said that she took to cigarettes by copying her father and that she would steal cigarettes that were half used from her father's ashtray. She had thought of giving up before but was never able to carry it through.

Mary found that she gradually became more breathless over time and was diagnosed with COPD five years ago. She was given an inhaler to be used whenever she felt breathless. This helped with her symptoms initially.

However, as time went on, she felt that she needed to use her rescue inhaler more and more. She was using it up to four times a day. On occasions, she would be using more than eight puffs of her inhaler in a day.

She returned to her doctor for help. Mary was started on regular inhalers for better control of her symptoms.

Unfortunately, Mary was not able to give up smoking. This was not helped by the fact that most of her family and friends also smoke. Everyone would smoke when there was a gathering of relatives or friends. It was also part of the social etiquette to smoke among her group of friends.

Mary became more breathless as the months went by and her breathing continued to decline. The medications did help with her breathing but they did not take away her breathlessness completely.

Mary knew that something had to be done. She felt that if her breathing were to continue to go downhill at this rate, she might soon not be able to breathe at all, even with the inhalers. She was determined to take a positive step forward and made a firm mental effort to stop smoking.

Mary has now managed to cut down her smoking to 10 cigarettes a day and is continuing to try hard to stop completely.

Comments on case study

Mary has moderate COPD that requires control with daily therapy. Her symptoms are currently on an even keel as the regular inhalers are keeping her airways opened. Unfortunately, with the ongoing insult to the lungs from the tobacco smoke, Mary's condition is likely to get worse.

It would be best if Mary could stop smoking altogether. This will not only slow down the decline in her lung function but also help reduce her risk of developing lung cancer.

Although smoking is a major risk factor for developing COPD and lung cancer, many smokers find it very hard to give up. The nicotine in cigarettes is a highly addictive compound, making giving up smoking a very difficult process indeed.

If you are struggling to give up, see your doctor who will be able to offer advice on how to stop. There are support and medications available that will help you cope with the early stages of nicotine withdrawal and craving.

Paul – severe COPD

Paul is 70 years old and this is his third admission to hospital this year with a flare-up of his COPD. He is getting very frustrated at having to come in to hospital so often. Each time he comes in and out of hospital, he feels that he is getting a little bit weaker.

His hospital stay also seems to get longer with each admission and subsequent chest infections seem harder to treat compared with the previous ones. At the same time, he is also frightened about being discharged home too soon, just in case he gets another flare-up and struggles to breathe.

Help is not easily at hand because he lives alone. Carers visit during the day but it is the nights that worry him most.

Paul is on a lot of medication for his COPD. He takes regular inhalers and tablet medications to help him breathe better. He also receives regular nebuliser therapy.

In addition, Paul has an oxygen concentrator at home that he uses to deliver continuous oxygen for more than 15 hours a day. Each day he has to take a fair amount of time to sort out his different medications and to work out the time of day that he needs to take them. He finds this is getting harder lately with his failing eyesight and his difficulty in concentrating.

Paul gets breathless very easily. Daily chores such as dressing and undressing or even just simply moving around the house will affect his breathing.

Paul tires easily and is no longer able to go upstairs. He has started to feel down and sometimes wonder whether life is worth living with the limitations and restrictions that are being imposed on him by his disabling COPD.

Comments on case study

Paul has severe COPD and is currently on maximum therapy. He is not able to do much without getting breathless. Paul is also starting to become depressed. The limitations that are created from living with severe COPD can be overwhelming. Paul is unable to do the simple things in life that we take for granted without struggling for breath.

Having COPD will make you more prone to develop chest infections. It is important to recognise infections early and treat them quickly to avoid a bad flare-up. However, you may find that, despite all the precautions that you take, you still end up with an infection. Do not despair, as people with COPD are generally more susceptible to developing repeated infections. Seek medical attention from your doctor to receive appropriate and prompt treatment.

You may feel discouraged and down because of your daily struggles with COPD. Stay positive and do not give in to desperation. It is totally understandable if you become depressed. This can be expected, because it is difficult to have to live with a chronic disabling condition.

It is important that you recognise depression early and seek medical help. Do not try to deal with it on your own.

Maintain a healthy lifestyle and diet. Always try to stay active and go outdoors when the weather permits. A little activity goes a long way in COPD. Try to develop a good social support network. Involve your relatives and friends in your daily life. Learn more about COPD. This will help you to cope better with it.

KEY POINTS

■ Smoking is the major cause of COPD

■ The symptoms of COPD can be relieved by medication

What is COPD?

How do we breathe?

Air enters the lungs through the nose and mouth. It then travels down the trachea or windpipe before going into the left and right lungs. The airways of the lung consist of the trachea, which then divides into two main tubes known as the left main bronchus and the right main bronchus.

The bronchial tubes then split further into smaller divisions known as bronchioles before finally reaching the alveolus or air sac. It is through the air sacs that air enters the bloodstream.

What is COPD?

COPD is a disabling condition affecting the lungs and involving irreversible lung damage, so that the lungs can no longer function at full capacity. COPD has been known by other names in the past such as chronic obstructive airway disease (COAD) or chronic obstructive lung disease (COLD). These terms are now obsolete.

The respiratory system

The airways (trachea, bronchi and bronchioles) and airspaces within the lungs supply oxygen to and remove carbon dioxide from the body.

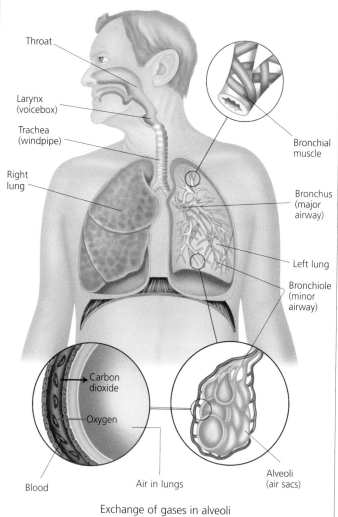

Throat

Larynx (voicebox)

Trachea (windpipe)

Right lung

Bronchial muscle

Bronchus (major airway)

Left lung

Bronchiole (minor airway)

Carbon dioxide

Oxygen

Blood

Air in lungs

Alveoli (air sacs)

Exchange of gases in alveoli

COPD comprises two related lung diseases:

- Chronic bronchitis
- Emphysema.

There is ongoing inflammation in the airways in COPD. The onset of breathlessness is gradual over time.

Chronic bronchitis

Chronic bronchitis results from inflammation and irritation of the airways in the lung. This causes airway narrowing, which can cause shortness of breath or wheezing. It is characterised by the presence of cough and phlegm production for more than three months in two consecutive years.

Emphysema

Air sacs deep within the lungs, where oxygen is absorbed into the bloodstream, are prone to damage from toxins such as tobacco smoke. Emphysema develops when the air sacs enlarge and are no longer able to function properly. This results in poor oxygen delivery to the blood circulation.

The chest muscles that are involved in breathing in people with emphysema have to work harder in order to sustain an adequate oxygen level in the blood. This contributes to breathlessness, which is made worse by the associated collapse in the surrounding airways caused by the loss of the lungs' natural elasticity as a consequence of lung tissue destruction. Air gets trapped in the lungs when the airways collapse during exhalation and this leads to hyperinflation of the lungs where the volume of the lungs becomes larger than normal.

Chronic bronchitis

In chronic bronchitis the airways are narrowed from inflammation and increased mucus secretions. This reduces the amount of air that passes through the lungs.

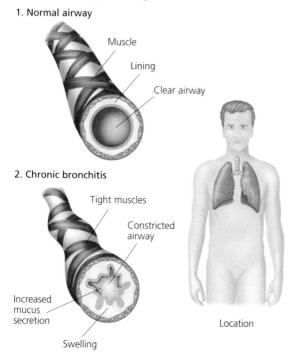

1. Normal airway

Muscle

Lining

Clear airway

2. Chronic bronchitis

Tight muscles

Constricted airway

Increased mucus secretion

Swelling

Location

The burden of COPD

COPD affects about three million people in the UK. It therefore places a tremendous burden on the health service and is the fourth most common cause of death worldwide. COPD also represents a considerable economic and social burden globally. The total estimated cost of COPD in the USA in 2002 was US$32.1 billion. In the UK, COPD accounted for more than £800 million

Emphysema

Emphysema develops when the alveoli (air sacs) are damaged by toxins. They become enlarged and no longer able to function properly.

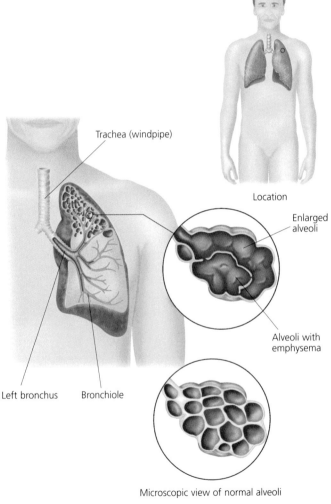

Location

Trachea (windpipe)

Enlarged alveoli

Alveoli with emphysema

Left bronchus

Bronchiole

Microscopic view of normal alveoli

The mechanics of breathing

To inhale air, muscles in the chest wall contract, lifting the ribs and pulling them outwards. The diaphragm moves downward enlarging the chest cavity further. Reduced air pressure in the lungs causes air to enter the lungs from outside. Breathing out reverses this.

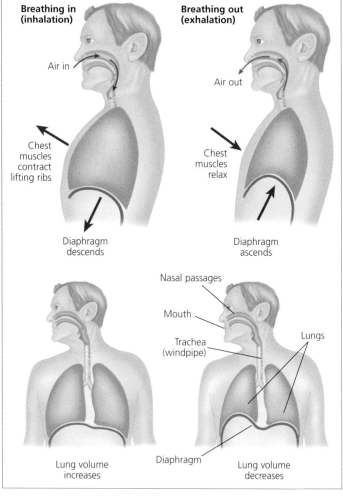

Breathing in (inhalation)

Air in

Chest muscles contract lifting ribs

Diaphragm descends

Breathing out (exhalation)

Air out

Chest muscles relax

Diaphragm ascends

Nasal passages

Mouth

Trachea (windpipe)

Lungs

Diaphragm

Lung volume increases

Lung volume decreases

in direct health-care costs in 2004 and this continues to rise annually.

Symptoms of COPD

- Many people get used to their COPD without realising it, especially in the early stages of the condition.

- You may find that you become tired easily when gardening or get out of breath when walking on an incline.

- People with COPD also tend to produce phlegm, particularly in the mornings.

- You may find that you always need to bring up phlegm by constantly coughing.

- You may also find it hard sometimes to shift phlegm from your lungs.

- The phlegm is usually clear in colour. Green or brown discoloration of thickened phlegm usually indicates an infection. Chest infection is common in people with COPD, especially during the winter months. It is important to recognise infection early and to seek medical treatment.

Causes of COPD
Smoking

Smoking is the main cause of COPD. It is estimated that smoking directly causes up to 90 per cent of COPD.

There are about 4,000 substances in tobacco smoke, of which 250 are classified as toxic matter and 60 are known to cause cancer in the body, such as in the bladder, cervix, kidneys, larynx or voicebox, lips, lungs, mouth, oesophagus or gullet, pancreas, stomach and throat.

Tobacco smoke damages the lungs. It also causes inflammation and irritation of the airways. Tar that is found in tobacco smoke injures and kills the cilia or tiny hairs that line the airways.

The cilia are like little brooms sweeping up dirt, germs and mucus in the airways. Smoking increases the susceptibility to developing chest infections as sticky tar covers and makes the cilia inefficient. Worsening breathlessness and a rapid decline in COPD may result with each, and subsequent, infection in the lungs.

If you are currently smoking, it is very important that you stop. This is the very best first step that you can take in battling this condition. You will also slow down the progression of the disease. Stopping smoking will not only halt the daily damage to your airways but it will also help your general well-being. You will start to notice an improvement in your complexion and your taste buds will jump back into life.

Remember that tobacco smoke can also affect those around a smoker. The detrimental effects of passive smoking are so overwhelming that the UK government outlawed smoking in public places throughout England on 1 July 2007. It is not enough simply to smoke outside the house because smoke particles have been shown to enter the house readily.

A smoker is 10 times more likely to die from COPD than a person who does not smoke. Both active and passive smoking are known to cause lung cancer and other serious medical problems such as heart disease and stroke.

People with COPD are particularly susceptible to the effects of tobacco smoke. Continuing to smoke even a little will significantly worsen the condition, leading to further deterioration.

Tobacco smoke damages cilia

Hair-like projections called cilia line the airways. Their function is to remove microbes and debris from the interior of the lungs.

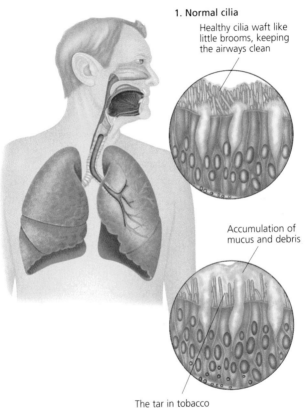

1. Normal cilia

Healthy cilia waft like little brooms, keeping the airways clean

Accumulation of mucus and debris

The tar in tobacco smoke compromises and kills cilia

2. Damaged cilia

The dangers of smoking

Both active and passive smoking are known to cause lung cancer and other serious medical problems. The illustration below shows the possible effects of smoking on the body.

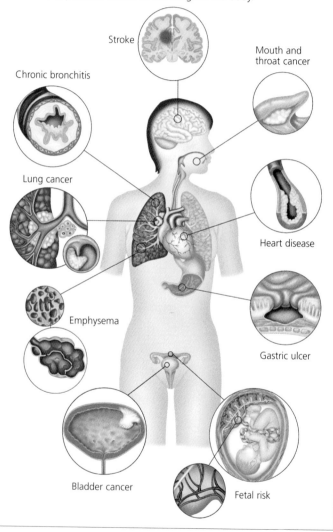

Stroke

Mouth and throat cancer

Chronic bronchitis

Lung cancer

Heart disease

Emphysema

Gastric ulcer

Bladder cancer

Fetal risk

Other causes of COPD

Alpha-1-antitrypsin deficiency

Tobacco smoke causes harm to the lungs by attracting inflammatory cells that release a substance or enzyme known as elastase. This enzyme breaks down elastin, which is an important structural component of lung tissue.

The lungs are protected from the potentially damaging effects of elastase through an inhibitor known as alpha-1-antitrypsin. By cancelling out the harmful effects of elastase, alpha-1-antitrypsin is able to protect the lungs from damage during infections and exposure to irritants such as tobacco smoke.

However, continued smoking will lead to substantial elastase being produced in high quantities, to such a level that the lungs' protective alpha-1-antitrypsin is no longer able to cope. Tobacco smoke in itself can also inactivate alpha-1-antitrypsin.

There is a hereditary genetic condition characterised by a defect in the body's ability to produce alpha-1-antitrypsin. This is known as alpha-1-antitrypsin deficiency. Normally the liver produces alpha-1-antitrypsin in the body, which then travels to the lungs via the bloodstream.

When a deficiency of alpha-1-antitrypsin occurs, the lungs are poorly protected from the destructive effects of elastase. This consequently leads to lung tissue damage and the development of emphysema.

Chest infections

COPD may also be more likely to occur in people who have had severe chest infections as children. Lung growth may be impaired by childhood chest infections and this, together with exposure to toxic agents such as tobacco smoke, increases the risk of developing COPD.

Bronchiectasis and chronic asthma

Bronchiectasis and chronic asthma may also lead to COPD. Bronchiectasis is lung damage characterised by enlarged and distended airways.

This causes ineffective phlegm clearance and repeated chest infections. In more than half of the people with bronchiectasis, the exact cause is never found. However, known causes for bronchiectasis include:

- inhalation of foreign objects such as peanuts, which block the bronchial tubes

- a weak immune system, which fights infection poorly

- severe indigestion with stomach acid getting into the lungs through backflow from the oesophagus (gullet)

- cilia that do not function properly, leading to ineffective clearance of phlegm

- a genetic condition known as cystic fibrosis, in which the bronchial tubes become clogged with thick and sticky mucus, resulting in constant inflammation and recurrent chest infections.

Asthma results from inflammation and narrowing in the airways. People with asthma tend to have a strong family history of asthma, eczema or allergies. Asthma is also more common in people who suffer from nose allergies.

This is because the nose and the lungs form part of the same passageway through which air travels into and out of the body, known collectively as the unified airway. Asthma also tends to affect people who have allergies to common inhaled airborne allergens such as house-dust mite, grass pollen, tree pollen, weed pollen, cat dander, dog dander and mould spores.

Allergies to common ingested food allergens such as wheat, egg white and peanuts may also cause asthma. Exposure to substances in the air such as environmental pollution and irritants found in the workplace can lead to asthma.

Asthma can also develop after chest infections including colds and flu. The symptoms in asthma may be very similar to those of COPD and sometimes it can be difficult to distinguish between the two conditions.

As a general rule of thumb, asthma tends to affect younger people who do not smoke whereas most older people with COPD either are current smokers or have smoked in the past.

Occupational exposures

COPD can also result from being exposed to chemical fumes and organic dusts, such as welding fumes, coal dust and cadmium. This is known as occupational exposure. The lungs are damaged as a result of inhalation of harmful compounds at work.

Other complications from COPD

COPD also affects other organs of the human body. The heart and lung function as one unit. Lung damage over time makes the blood vessels in the lungs constrict and harden. This causes the blood pressure in the lungs to increase and makes it harder for the heart to pump blood to it. This is known as pulmonary hypertension, and may subsequently lead to poor functioning of the heart, otherwise known as heart failure.

If your heart is affected, you will find that you start to retain fluid in your body and that your ankles start

Breathlessness

Breathlessness is a frequently occurring symptom of heart failure.

Lungs

Capillary network

Alveoli (air sacs)

Fluid collects in airspaces of lungs

Excessive fluid flows out of blood into lung tissue

Inside of lung

Capillary

to swell. It becomes more difficult for you to lie flat on your bed because you require more and more pillows to sleep in order to be more comfortable.

On some occasions, you find yourself waking up in the middle of the night gasping for breath. See your doctor if you start to develop these symptoms because your heart may have been affected.

Swollen ankles

Swollen ankles can be a symptom of heart failure.

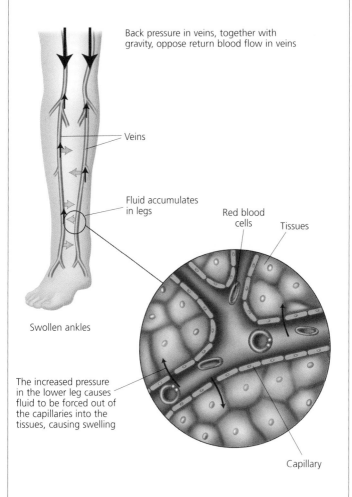

Back pressure in veins, together with gravity, oppose return blood flow in veins

Veins

Fluid accumulates in legs

Red blood cells

Tissues

Swollen ankles

The increased pressure in the lower leg causes fluid to be forced out of the capillaries into the tissues, causing swelling

Capillary

Outlook for people with COPD

There is currently no cure for COPD. People with COPD will have to live with the condition for the rest of their lives. Nevertheless, there are various treatments and support available, which may help. The main aim of these approaches is to alleviate symptoms while reducing flare-ups.

KEY POINTS

- COPD can be very disabling; there is currently no known cure but appropriate treatment and support will help

- Smoking damages the lungs and is the most common cause of COPD; it is very important that you stop if you are currently smoking

- COPD places a tremendous burden on the health service both locally and globally

Diagnosis

Symptoms of COPD
COPD can affect people in many different ways.

People with COPD may experience shortness of breath with or without wheezing. In some, breathlessness may be present only on exertion. Others may struggle for breath just by carrying out normal activities that most of us take for granted such as dressing and undressing or simply walking around the house. Shortness of breath can also be constant in people with COPD and may be present even at rest.

Some people may not even be breathless at all but have constant coughs and phlegm production. Others may get symptoms only when they catch flu or a chest infection during the winter months.

Other effects of COPD
It is now recognised that COPD may lead to feelings of anxiety, tiredness, frustration and even depression. It is therefore important to be active in both mind and body. Maintaining a positive frame of mind and a positive outlook will help to achieve this.

Pattern of development

COPD usually creeps up unnoticed and comes on gradually over several years. The age of onset is usually above 35 years. People with COPD may not notice that they have symptoms of the condition early on, because the body is able to adjust naturally. However, with time, and the normal ageing process, this delicate balance is tipped. The body can no longer compensate and symptoms such as breathlessness will begin to surface when climbing stairs or hurrying.

As the condition progresses, shortness of breath may be present even while walking on the flat. In severe cases, the normal activities of daily living such as changing clothes or moving about the house may become difficult.

There are several screening questionnaires available to assess whether a person may have COPD or not.

Do I have COPD?

If two or more of the following statements are true for you, and you are over 35 years old, it is advisable that you see your doctor.

- I have been smoking for many years.
- I have had bouts of 'asthma' or 'bronchitis'.
- I have a chronic cough or heavy phlegm.
- I have morning 'smoker's cough'.
- My colds last for weeks, not days, and I have at least one prolonged episode of 'bronchitis' every winter.
- I frequently feel breathless during an ordinary activity – I often put this down to just being 'out of shape'.
- My cough has changed – it feels shallower, as though something is stuck inside my chest.
- I feel that there has been a change in my breathing.

The box on page 26 gives an example of a simple and straightforward questionnaire developed by the Canadian Lung Association.

Severity

To assess the severity of COPD, a scale has been devised by the UK Medical Research Council (MRC). It is a simple standardised tool used to gauge the severity of COPD. The scale ranges from grade 1 to grade 5 according to the degree of breathlessness related to activities.

MRC breathlessness scale

Grade	Degree of breathlessness related to activities
1	Not troubled by breathlessness except on strenuous exercise
2	Short of breath when hurrying or walking up a slight hill
3	Walks slower than contemporaries on level ground because of breathlessness, or has to stop for breath when walking at own pace
4	Stops for breath after walking about 100 metres or after a few minutes on level ground
5	Too breathless to leave the house, or breathless when dressing or undressing

Investigation

Various investigations can be performed in order to establish whether you have COPD or other chest problems such as asthma or bronchiectasis. Simple tests can be performed in your GP surgery by either the doctor or the nurse. More complicated tests are carried out in hospital and are usually requested by the chest specialist.

Spirometry

A blowing test is usually performed to diagnose COPD. This is known as spirometry and can easily be carried out in your GP surgery.

You will be required to blow as hard as you can into a machine through a mouthpiece. It will give important information as to whether your airways are narrowed.

Spirometry

Spirometry measures not only how fast air can be blown out, but also the amount of air blown out with each breath.

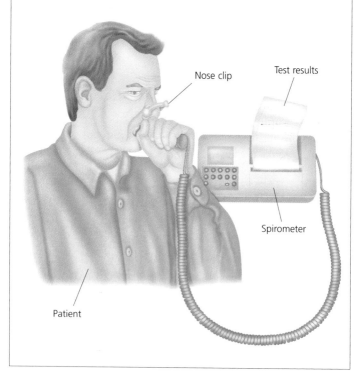

Nose clip

Test results

Spirometer

Patient

Measurements obtained from the spirometer include the following:

- The amount of air that you can blow out in one second, known as the forced expiratory volume in one second or FEV_1

- The total amount of air that you can blow out in one breath, known as the forced vital capacity or FVC

- The proportion of air that you can blow out in one second, known as the FEV_1/FVC ratio.

Your airways are generally considered to be narrowed if your FEV_1 is reduced and the FEV_1/FVC ratio is less than 0.7.

Lung function test

Sometimes a more comprehensive test is required. It is known as a full lung function test. This test is usually performed in a hospital lung laboratory. Your doctor will refer you to a chest specialist in the hospital for this. It will enable the hospital doctor to make a correct diagnosis.

In addition to obtaining the basic measurements of the spirometer such as FEV_1, FVC and FEV_1/FVC ratio, the full lung function test also measures the following:

- The volume of air contained in the lungs after a full inhalation, known as the total lung capacity or TLC

- The remaining volume of air in the lungs after full exhalation, known as the residual volume or RV

- How efficiently the lungs transfer oxygen from the air into the bloodstream, known as the carbon monoxide transfer factor or T_{LCO} and the carbon monoxide transfer coefficient or K_{CO}.

Lung function test

A full lung function test is usually undertaken in a hospital lung laboratory. It will give your doctor very comprehensive data about the health of your lungs.

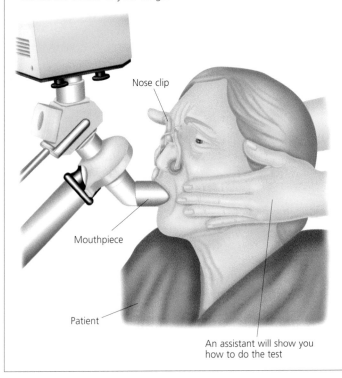

Nose clip

Mouthpiece

Patient

An assistant will show you how to do the test

Usually, in people with COPD, the TLC and RV are increased as a result of air trapping and the T_{LCO} and K_{CO} are reduced as a result of emphysema.

Chest X-ray

A chest X-ray may also be useful and is usually taken in the radiology department of the hospital. There is virtually no risk involved because the dose of radiation

Chest X-ray

X-rays are electromagnetic rays that can penetrate soft tissues, but are absorbed by bones or opaque contrast media. They can be very useful for diagnosing internal disorders.

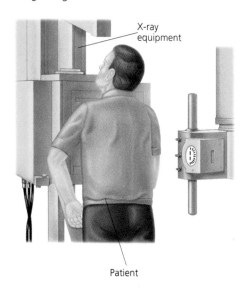

X-ray equipment

Patient

from a chest X-ray is very small, and equivalent to about 0.25% of the yearly natural background radiation that we receive from exposure to cosmic rays and radioactive minerals in the ground.

In COPD, the lungs are usually expanded more than normal and lung hyperinflation caused by air trapping may be readily seen on the chest X-ray. It is also important to have a chest X-ray when people with COPD are unwell with chest infections. This is to look for pneumonia, which is a serious infection of the lungs. The affected areas that are infected in the lungs should be visible on the chest X-ray and this would usually give an indication of the severity of the pneumonia.

Laboratory tests

A sample of your phlegm may also be required. You will usually be given a pot by either your doctor or chest specialist for you to collect the specimen, which can then be handed over at your GP surgery or the hospital depending on which location is more convenient for you. This is to assess whether there is any infection present in the lungs.

A positive culture result from the phlegm sample usually indicates an infection. A course of antibiotics may be required to treat the infection. You may not require antibiotic treatment if the culture result is negative, which may indicate that the infection is viral rather than a bacteria. Antibiotics work only in bacterial infections because they are not effective against viruses.

CT scan

Computed tomography, also known as CT, of the lung is usually reserved for cases when a further detailed examination is required. It is a painless test and simply requires you to lie on a couch, which then slides forwards and backwards through a doughnut-shaped hole while pictures are taken.

A CT scan may be used for further study of an abnormality picked up on the chest X-ray. It may also be used to investigate suspected lung cancer. CT scan can be performed only on the request of the chest specialist after consultation. This is to ensure that the number of times that a CT scan is undertaken is kept to a necessary minimum because the radiation dose is about 80 times that of a chest X-ray.

Computed tomography (CT)

Computed tomography fires X-rays through the body at different angles. The X-rays are picked up by receivers and the information analysed by a computer to create a picture of the body.

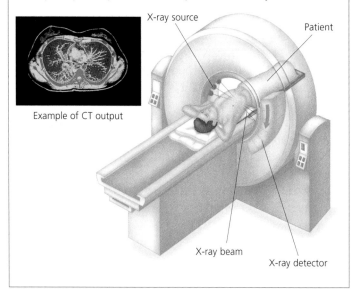

Example of CT output

X-ray source

Patient

X-ray beam

X-ray detector

Flare-up

From time to time, people with COPD will find that their condition worsens; this is known as a 'flare-up'. A flare-up is also commonly known as an 'exacerbation'. It usually occurs during the winter when the weather is cold. Most people find that their COPD is usually worse at this time of the year.

A flare-up is commonly caused by a chest infection, although this may not necessarily be the sole reason. For instance, sensitivity to cold air leading to narrowing of the airways can also lead to a flare-up.

Bacteria and viruses

During the winter there are more infections around. Common infections during this period include flu and pneumonia. Flu is caused by the influenza virus and pneumonia by pneumococcal bacteria.

Antibiotics will work only against bacterial infection because they are useless against viral infection. Viruses are usually dealt with by the body's own immune system. However, sometimes a viral infection may be so overwhelming that it weakens the body's immunity and predisposes the lungs to catching an infection known as a secondary bacterial infection; this can usually be treated with a course of antibiotics.

Symptoms during a flare-up

During a flare-up, you may find that you are more breathless than usual. You may be struggling for breath and your medications may not be working as well. You may also find that you are wheezing or coughing up more phlegm than usual, and feel generally unwell and weak or even have a fever.

It is important that you see a doctor during a flare-up. Your doctor will be able to assess you and suggest appropriate treatment. If your flare-up cannot be managed at home, your doctor will usually recommend that you be admitted to hospital.

Do not be discouraged or feel apprehensive about it. Many people with COPD who have a flare-up are admitted to hospital. This is to ensure that further investigations such as a check on the blood oxygen level or a chest X-ray are carried out. Appropriate management may then be tailored accordingly.

Making plans to deal with flare-ups

Your doctor may wish to draw up an action plan with you. This usually involves consultation with your doctor to discuss a course of action that you may wish to take should you have a flare-up or feel that a flare-up may be on the horizon.

Sometimes, if you are confident about managing your COPD, and if you are agreeable to a pre-discussed plan, your doctor may supply you with some antibiotics and oral corticosteroids to have at home with you.

On pages 38–43 there are two excellent examples of COPD action plans by the Australian Lung Foundation and the US National Jewish Medical and Research Center.

When you feel that your COPD is getting bad or when you have an infection, your doctor may suggest that you take an antibiotic and a corticosteroid course. This is so that you can treat the infection more quickly and hopefully prevent a full-blown flare-up requiring hospital admission.

It is not always easy to distinguish between a bacterial and a viral infection on clinical grounds and on balance it is usually safer to treat the infection with antibiotics during a COPD flare-up. Some antibiotics have also been shown to have anti-inflammatory properties in addition to their anti-bacterial activity, and the former may justify their use in a flare-up regardless of whether it is caused by a bacterial or viral infection, bearing in mind that a secondary bacterial infection may stem from a viral infection.

However, if you do not respond to the treatment, it is very important that you see your doctor immediately.

The differences between bacteria and viruses

Both viruses and bacteria are microscopic organisms that can enter the body cells.

1. Viruses

Viruses are minute organisms. They are parasitic in that they are dependent on nutrients inside cells to survive and reproduce. A virus is very simple, consisting of a strand of genetic material covered by protein.

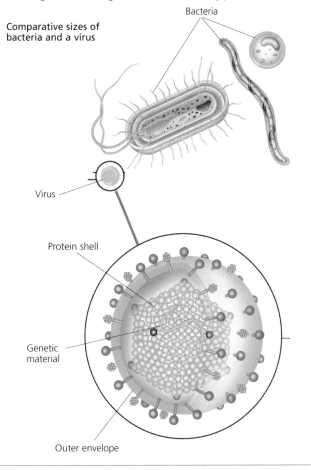

Comparative sizes of bacteria and a virus

Bacteria

Virus

Protein shell

Genetic material

Outer envelope

The differences between bacteria and viruses (contd)

2. Bacteria

There are three principal forms of bacteria – rod shaped, curved and spherical. Rod-shaped or curved bacteria are able to move independently using the flagellum – a whip-like structure. If bacteria produce disease they are called pathogenic.

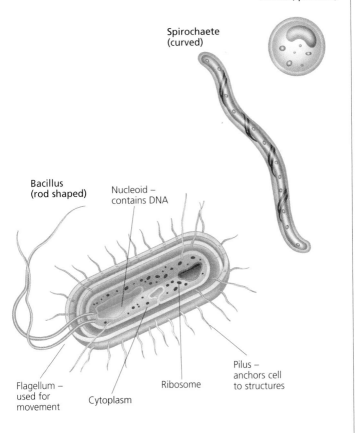

Coccus (spherical)

Spirochaete (curved)

Bacillus (rod shaped)

Nucleoid – contains DNA

Flagellum – used for movement

Cytoplasm

Ribosome

Pilus – anchors cell to structures

COPD action plan

Patient Name:	Date of birth:
GP Name:	GP Phone:
	After Hours Phone:
Consultant Name:	Consultant Phone:
Outreach/Community Nurse Phone:	Ambulance Phone:

USUAL TREATMENT WHEN STABLE:

Best FEV_1 _____ Best FVC _____

Room air O_2 saturation _____ % □ CO_2 Retainer

Oxygen: l/min _____ _____ hours/day

MY REGULAR MEDICATION/S	STRENGTH	DOSE	ROUTE pMDI + SPACER / DPI / NEBULISER / ORAL	HOW OFTEN
1				
2				
3				
4				
5				
6				

MODERATE ATTACK
(UNWELL BUT NOT SEVERE)

- More wheezy/breathless
- Increased cough and sputum
- Change in colour of sputum
- Loss of appetite/sleep
- Taking more reliever medication than usual

- NOTIFY GP OR OTHER
  HEALTH PROFESSIONAL

- Eat small amounts more often
- Use controlled breathing techniques
- Use a huff and puff cough to clear secretions
- Use anxiety/stress management techniques

EXTRA RELIEVER	STRENGTH	DOSE	ROUTE	HOW OFTEN
1				
2				
3				

PREDNISOLONE (reducing schedule)	STRENGTH	TABS/DOSE	DAYS
start			
then			
then			
then			

ANTIBIOTIC	STRENGTH	DOSE	ROUTE	HOW OFTEN
1				
2				

SEVERE ATTACK
- Call ambulance – 999
- Show them this plan and say you
  have severe COPD

My Symptoms:
- Unable to perform normal activites, e.g. dress, bathe
- Fever / chills
- Increased swelling of ankles
- Extremely short of breath

NAME: SIGNATURE: DATE:

Self-management plan
Action to take when you experience
increased symptoms

Breathing

Green zone

1 You are able to breathe without difficulty while doing your usual activities.

Continue with your usual activities.

Exercise as directed by your doctor.

Take your medications as ordered by your doctor.

Yellow zone

2 You have more shortness of breath, wheezing or coughing than usual.

You have an unexplained increase or decrease in weight along with swelling in your feet or ankles.

Take nebulised treatment or your rescue inhaler as ordered by your doctor.

Use pursed-lip breathing and relaxation exercises.

Increase your medications ONLY if directed by your doctor.

Check your oxygen equipment to see if it works right.

Check your saturation if you have pulse oximetry.

Increase oxygen ONLY as ordered by your doctor.

Start oral corticosteroids ONLY if directed by your doctor.

Call your doctor/respiratory nurse if not better in 1–2 hours.

Red zone

3 You are having a lot of trouble breathing.

You have increased trouble breathing at rest or suddenly need to sleep on more pillows or in a chair.

Call your doctor NOW

Call 999 if you are unable to talk to the doctor or nurse right away OR go to the nearest accident and emergency department (A&E).

Follow actions in yellow zone above.

Go to A&E if you are frightened by not being able to breathe.

Self-management plan
Action to take when you experience
increased symptoms

Sputum

Green zone

1 Your sputum is
  clear/white
  and easy to
  cough up.

  You have a small
  amount of sputum.

Continue with your usual activities.

Exercise as directed by your doctor.

Take your medications as ordered by your doctor.

Yellow zone

2 Your sputum is
  thicker or stickier
  than usual.

  Your sputum is
  green, yellow or
  brown for more
  than 12 hours.

  You develop a fever
  above 38°C.

Increase fluids (non-caffeine drinks) if no fluid limits.

Call your doctor if on fluid restriction.

Start other medications to thin mucus if ordered by
  doctor.

Use flutter valve/chest percussion/huff coughing as
  ordered.

Take nebulised treatment or rescue inhaler as
  ordered by your doctor.

Start antibiotics if ordered by your doctor.

Increase oxygen if directed by doctor.

Call doctor to inform about sputum changes.

Call your respiratory nurse.

Red zone

3 You are having a
  lot of trouble
  coughing up any
  sputum.

  You have blood in
  your sputum.

  You may have chest
  pain.

Call your doctor NOW.

Call 999 if you are unable to talk to the doctor or
  nurse right away OR go to the nearest A&E.

Follow actions in yellow zone above.

Self-management plan
Action to take when you experience
increased symptoms

Thinking

Green zone

1 You are able to think clearly

Continue with your usual activities.

Exercise as directed by your doctor.

Take your medications as ordered by your doctor.

Yellow zone

2 You are having trouble concentrating.

You are more forgetful and restless.

Check your oxygen system to see if it works right.

Check your saturation if you have pulse oximetry.

Increase oxygen ONLY if directed by doctor.

Do pursed-lip breathing and relaxation exercises.

Take nebulised treatment or rescue inhaler as ordered by your doctor.

Call doctor/respiratory nurse if not better in 1–2 hours.

Red zone

3 You are very confused, have slurred speech or feel like you are going to faint.

Call 999 if you have fainted or have slurred speech.

Call your doctor NOW if you are confused or feel like you are going to faint.

Call 999 if you are unable to talk to the doctor or nurse right away OR go to the nearest A&E.

Follow actions in yellow zone above.

Self-management plan
Action to take when you experience
increased symptoms

Energy

Green zone

1 You can do your usual activities without tiring.

Continue with your usual activities.

Exercise as directed by your doctor.

Take your medications as ordered by your doctor.

Yellow zone

2 You are tired and not able to finish usual activities without resting.

You have a feeling that in general your health has worsened.

You have new difficulty sleeping.

You have morning headaches, dizzy spells or restlessness.

You wake up feeling very tired or are tired by late afternoon.

Pace yourself and limit your activities.

Use pursed-lip breathing.

Check your oxygen system to see if it works right.

Check your saturation if you have pulse oximetry.

Increase oxygen ONLY if directed by your doctor.

Start oral corticosteroids ONLY if directed by your doctor.

Call doctor/respiratory nurse.

Red zone

3 You are not able to do any activities.

You are very drowsy.

You are difficult to arouse (wake up).

Call 999 if you feel like you are going to faint or are suddenly very confused.

Call your doctor/respiratory nurse NOW.

Follow actions in yellow zone above.

Go to A&E if you are frightened by how tired or drowsy you feel.

Work with your doctor

You must also make sure that any plan to self-manage your COPD in the event of it getting worse needs to be fully discussed and agreed by your doctor first.

You must not at any stage take matters into your own hands and start treating any infection or flare-up yourself. You may know a lot about your COPD, but your doctor is independent and trained to recognise any warning signs of a serious nature.

KEY POINTS

■ COPD affects different people in different ways

■ Objective confirmation through a blowing test such as spirometry will usually be required in order to diagnose COPD

■ It is important to recognise and treat a flare-up promptly, which could help to avoid a hospital admission

Drug treatment

Types of treatment

The main aim of treatment is to relieve breathlessness. It does not reverse or cure the underlying condition but may improve symptoms and reduce flare-ups.

There are several forms of treatment available divided into two categories:

1 Inhaled therapy

2 Oral therapy.

Inhaled therapy

Inhalers can come in a variety of different devices. The number of times that you need to take a particular medication can also vary. It is therefore important that you are familiar with the medications that have been prescribed for you.

Be safe. Always get help without delay if you are uncertain or in doubt about how to use your medications. People who may offer assistance and advice include your:

- doctor
- practice nurse
- pharmacist.

Inhaled therapy is broadly divided into two main groups:

- reliever medication
- preventer medication.

Reliever medication
Reliever or rescue medications can provide immediate relief from breathlessness or wheezing. There are no fixed times to take them. They should be taken as and when the need arises.

Preventer medication
Preventer medications keep the airways opened and help control inflammation in the lungs. They need to be taken regularly to be effective. Typically they are taken twice a day every day. They can help prevent flare-ups and reduce the use of reliever medication.

Class of medication
Corticosteroids
Corticosteroids are commonly mistaken for anabolic steroids abused by some athletes and body builders. Anabolic steroids are very different from the corticosteroids used in COPD.

Inhaled corticosteroids are used as preventer medication. They treat inflammation in the airways by inhibiting substances and cells that are involved in the

Inhaler therapy

Inhaling a drug is the most effective treatment for the prevention and relief of COPD symptoms. The inhaler distributes the drug rapidly through the airways for instant relief of symptoms.

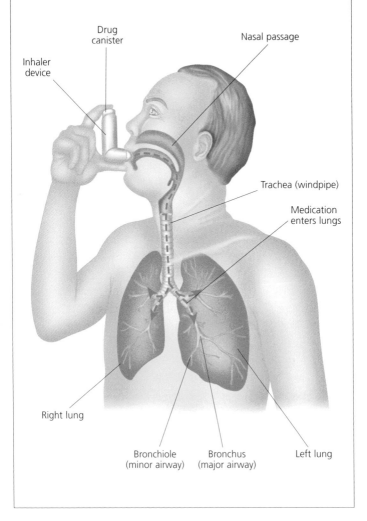

Drug canister

Nasal passage

Inhaler device

Trachea (windpipe)

Medication enters lungs

Right lung

Bronchiole (minor airway)

Bronchus (major airway)

Left lung

inflammatory process. They are usually taken twice daily on a regular basis.

Inhaled corticosteroids may not be necessary if you have only mild COPD or suffer from very infrequent flare-ups. Examples of inhaled corticosteroids include:

- beclometasone (AeroBec)

- budesonide (Pulmicort)

- fluticasone (Flixotide).

Side effects
There are a few possible side effects with inhaled corticosteroids. They can cause thrush in the mouth or throat. Sometimes voice hoarseness or a sore throat may develop.

These side effects can generally be prevented by regular mouth rinsing after each morning and evening treatment. Recently it has been increasingly recognised that there may be the potential risk of developing osteoporosis in people who are receiving high doses of inhaled corticosteroids.

This risk can be minimised by your doctor who will make sure that you are receiving only the lowest possible dose of inhaled corticosteroids that is effective for you. You can also help reduce the risk by taking simple steps such as regular exercise and ensuring that you are receiving enough calcium in your diet to keep your bones strong and healthy.

Beta-2 agonists
There are two groups of inhaled beta-2 agonists:

- short acting

- long acting.

They stimulate beta-2 receptors on the smooth muscle cells in the lining of the airways. This causes the muscle cells to relax, which then opens up the airways.

Short-acting beta-2 agonists are used as reliever medication. They act quickly to relieve breathlessness or wheezing. There are taken when the need arises and their effects last for around four hours. Examples of short-acting beta-2 agonists include:

- salbutamol (Ventolin)
- terbutaline (Bricanyl).

Long-acting beta-2 agonists keep the airways opened for up to 12 hours. They are used as preventer medication. They are usually taken twice a day. Examples of long-acting beta-2 agonists include:

- formoterol (Oxis)
- salmeterol (Serevent).

Side effects
The two side effects that they commonly cause are tremors and a faster than normal heart beat when taken in excess.

Anticholinergics
There are two forms of inhaled anticholinergics:

- short acting
- long acting.

They block receptors known as muscarinic receptors in the lungs. These receptors cause narrowing of the airways and blocking them allows the airways to open up.

Short-acting anticholinergics act quickly and can relieve breathlessness for up to 6 hours. They are usually used four times daily. Examples of short-acting anticholinergics are:

- ipratropium (Atrovent).

Long-acting anticholinergics can help keep the airways open for up to 24 hours. They are used once daily. An example of a long-acting anticholinergic is tiotropium (Spiriva).

Side effects
The two most common side effects are causing a dry mouth and leaving a bad taste.

Combination inhalers
Manufacturers of inhalers have also combined different classes of medications into a single inhaler. This is much more convenient and reduces the number of inhalers required.

Examples of combination inhalers are:

- Combivent (ipratropium plus salbutamol)
- Seretide (fluticasone plus salmeterol)
- Symbicort (budesonide plus formoterol).

Types of inhaler devices
There are numerous inhaler devices available. Your doctor should usually assess whether you are able to use such a device before prescribing the inhaler. It is important that you are familiar with your inhaler device. Your practice nurse or pharmacist may also be able to help.

Different types of inhaler devices deliver different forms of medication.

Pressurised metered-dose inhalers

A pressurised metered-dose inhaler (pMDI) delivers medication in an aerosol form. Good coordination in pressing the inhaler and breathing in the aerosol is required.

This device may not be suitable if you have severe arthritis of the hands. If you have poor coordination, then the use of a spacer with the pMDI may be tried. A spacer can also enable better delivery of medication into the lungs. Alternatively, a breath-activated pMDI may be used. This works automatically when you breathe in, so there is no need to push a button.

Dry powder inhalers

A dry powder inhaler (DPI) delivers medication in powder form. Some people prefer this type of inhaler to the pMDI because they dislike the feel of the aerosol hitting the back of the throat. Others are more comfortable with the pMDI compared with the DPI because they are unable to feel the dry powder during inhalation and thus do not have the reassurance that they are actually receiving the medication. Personal preference ultimately determines the choice of inhaler device.

There is no coordination needed in using the inhaler device because you are simply required to take a deep breath once the inhaler is activated. Activation is usually by hand through a simple clicking mechanism in the device, which releases the medication ready for inhalation. The medication may be contained within the device itself or you may be required to insert a capsule containing the dry powder.

Nebulisers

A nebuliser delivers medication in vapour form. Liquid medication is converted into a fine mist, which is then breathed in through a mask or mouthpiece. It is usually used during a flare-up in hospital. Nebulisers can allow for higher doses of medication to be conveniently delivered to the lungs. It may also be useful for people who are unable to use inhaler devices.

Colour coding

You may have noticed that your inhalers not only come in different shapes and sizes, but are also of many different colours. Blue and shades of blue have been traditionally chosen to represent reliever medications. Preventer medications on the other hand are represented by different shades of brown.

There are also many other colours that can be found for different inhalers such as grey, green, purple and red. Although some manufacturers of inhalers adopt the standard colour coding, there are others who do not because they are not required by law to follow a set colour code.

Inhaler technique

The correct technique when using an inhaler is very important. This is to ensure that the correct amount of medication is delivered to your lungs. If you are unable to use your inhaler properly, then there is a chance that very little or none of the medication from your inhaler is being breathed into your lungs.

For a standard pMDI device, the following inhaler technique should be followed. As with all inhalers, it is very important that, in the first instance, someone such as your doctor, practice nurse or pharmacist shows you

How nebulisers work

The nebuliser is a simple air compressor. It bubbles air through a solution of the drug, generating a mist, which is inhaled through either a mask or a mouthpiece.

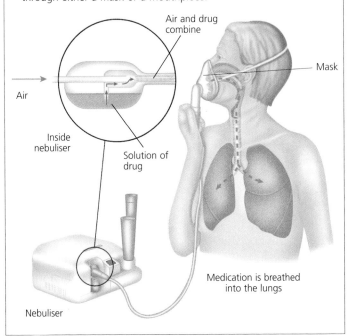

Air and drug combine

Mask

Air

Inside nebuliser

Solution of drug

Medication is breathed into the lungs

Nebuliser

the correct technique. Nothing is better than a real-life demonstration of the proper inhaler technique:

- Remove the cap from the pMDI.

- Give it a gentle shake to ensure a thorough mix of the pMDI contents.

- Exhale and breathe out as much as you possibly can.

- Put the pMDI in your mouth and start slowly to breathe in.

- Press the pMDI about two seconds after you have started breathing in slowly.

- Continue breathing in for as long as you can, preferably for 10 seconds.

- Now hold your breath for as long as you can manage, 10 seconds if possible.

- Exhale and breathe out slowly.

- Repeat the process if you require another puff of the pMDI.

- Remember to replace the cap when you have finished and store your pMDI in a safe place.

- Now rinse your mouth thoroughly.

Using a spacer

Using the pMDI correctly requires practice and good coordination. Not everyone will be able to use the pMDI properly. A spacer may be used along with a pMDI to help delivery of the medication. Coordination is not required when using a spacer. Remember the following as well when using a spacer with your pMDI:

- Press the pMDI to deliver one puff into the spacer.

- Breathe in slowly and deeply.

- Hold your breath for as long as you can, preferably for about 10 seconds.

- Breathe out away from the spacer.

- Now repeat by breathing in and holding your breath once again as above.

Spacer devices

These allow the patient to concentrate on breathing in the medication rather than having to coordinate inhaling and pressing the inhaler button at the same time.

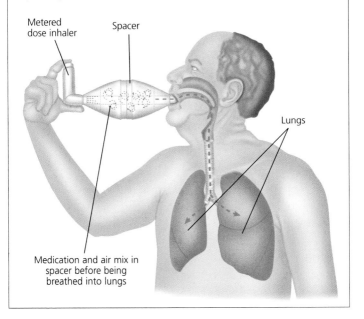

Metered dose inhaler

Spacer

Lungs

Medication and air mix in spacer before being breathed into lungs

- You should take two breaths for each puff of your pMDI.

- Do not press more than one puff of the pMDI at any one time into the spacer.

- Giving more than one puff from the pMDI into the spacer will cause the aerosols to bind together. This will affect the amount of medication that is delivered to your lungs. It will also cause the aerosols to stick to the inside of the spacer. As a result, the medication delivered may be less than intended.

The spacer should be washed once a month using mild detergent and allowed to dry in air. You should avoid more frequent cleaning because it will generate electrostatic charges that may interfere with delivery of the medication. Your spacer should be replaced with a new one once every 6 to 12 months.

Oral therapy

There are several oral medications available that are taken by mouth in tablet form. They are usually given in addition to inhaled therapy.

Class
Corticosteroids
Oral corticosteroids are used mainly during a flare-up. They control inflammation of the lungs and may help in hastening recovery.

Side effects
There are numerous possible side effects when taking oral corticosteroids, as they are absorbed into the bloodstream. Common side effects when taken short term include upset stomach, weight gain and trouble sleeping.

When taken long term, they can cause weakening of the immune system, thinning of the skin and brittle bones. Regular treatment with oral corticosteroids is therefore best avoided and should be reserved for flare-ups only.

There are, however, a small number of people who do use oral corticosteroids on a daily basis. This is usually to help with severe disabling COPD. Complete or sudden withdrawal of oral corticosteroids in people who are dependent on them may lead to ill health, flare-ups and deterioration in breathing. Additional medications to prevent bone thinning will be necessary if oral corticosteroids are taken long term.

An example of an oral corticosteroid is prednisolone.

Methylxanthines

Methylxanthines may be used in addition to inhaler medication. They inhibit substances known as phosphodiesterases, which are enzymes involved in the inflammatory process in the body and by doing so help reduce inflammation in the airways.

They need to be taken daily and may help with breathing. Regular blood tests will be required. This is to ensure that you are receiving the correct dose and to minimise unwanted side effects. An example of a methylxanthine is theophylline (Phyllocontin).

Side effects

They may cause nausea, vomiting and irregular heartbeats. When receiving this medication, you will need to have regular blood tests to check the levels of the medication in your body. It is important that you are receiving the correct dose because too high a level will lead to toxic effects and too low a level will not allow the medication to work properly.

Mucolytics

Mucolytics may also be prescribed. They loosen the phlegm in the lungs by making it less thick and sticky. This makes the phlegm easier to cough up. They may also improve breathlessness and help lessen chest infections by reducing the amount of phlegm. They are usually taken two to four times a day. Mucolytics include:

- carbocisteine (Mucodyne)

- mecysteine (Visclair).

Side effects
Mucolytics can cause a mild stomach upset and rash.

Antibiotics
Antibiotics may be used during a flare-up because they kill bacteria by interfering with their ability to form cell walls. Antibiotics can also prevent bacteria from multiplying.

They are not effective against viral infections. Antibiotics should not be used routinely to prevent infections because this may cause antibiotic resistance in bacteria and may lead to the development of so-called superbugs, which are immune to a multitude of routine antibiotics. Examples of antibiotics are:

- amoxicillin (Amoxil)

- clarithromycin (Klaricid).

Side effects
Antibiotics can cause a rash, diarrhoea, nausea and vomiting.

Antidepressants
Antidepressants may be prescribed to help with anxiety and depression related to COPD. They slow the breakdown of chemicals in the brain known as neurotransmitters. They may improve mood and enable relaxation. They are usually taken once daily. Examples of antidepressants are:

- citalopram (Cipramil)

- paroxetine (Seroxat).

Side effects
Antidepressants can cause nausea, vomiting and headache.

Anti-phosphodiesterases
Newer anti-phosphodiesterases such as phosphodiesterase-4 inhibitors are currently in the late stages of clinical trials. They inhibit a specific subtype of phosphodiesterase known as phosphodiesterase-4. They reduce inflammation in the airways and may help with breathlessness. Examples of phosphodiesterase-4 inhibitors are:

- roflumilast (Daxas)

- cilomilast (Ariflo).

Side effects
Phosphodiesterase-4 inhibitors can cause nausea, headache and diarrhoea.

KEY POINTS

■ The many different types of medications and devices available for treating COPD can be confusing

■ It is important that you are given appropriate instructions and tuition with regard to using your medication correctly by your prescriber

■ Reliever medication will provide immediate relief for breathlessness and is used when the need arises

■ Preventer medication will not act immediately and is taken daily in order to sustain benefit

Non-drug treatment

Oxygen therapy

Oxygen may be prescribed by the chest specialist during a flare-up where it may help with breathlessness. The airways may become narrower and the lungs more inflamed at the time of a flare-up and, as a result, less air enters the lungs with poorer oxygen delivery to the body.

Oxygen therapy can thus help boost the body's oxygen level during this period. Most people do not require oxygen once they leave hospital because their lungs heal and recover after appropriate treatment.

Some people with COPD will require oxygen at home. Oxygen can be used either continuously or when the need arises.

It is important that you first undergo appropriate and thorough assessment in hospital before receiving oxygen therapy. This is because oxygen therapy may not be suitable for everyone with COPD.

A referral to a chest specialist is required before oxygen can be prescribed for home use. Oxygen therapy is currently provided through the UK National Health Service (NHS) following recommendation from the chest specialist.

A blood test known as an arterial blood gas will be required. This test will give a measure of the oxygen and carbon dioxide levels in your blood.

The sample is usually taken from the radial artery in your wrist, where your pulse is felt. The test is more uncomfortable than a normal blood test. Pressure will have to be applied to the artery for at least five minutes after the test to avoid too much bruising.

Arterial blood gas sampling

Arterial blood is oxygenated blood flowing directly from the heart; analysis of arterial blood can determine the chemistry of the blood before it is used by the tissues.

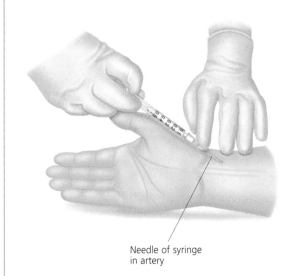

Needle of syringe
in artery

Oxygen cannot be prescribed for people who continue to smoke. This is because of the dangers of causing an explosion or a serious fire. In order to minimise the risk, you must ensure that no one around you smokes either.

Once a chest specialist has decided that you require oxygen therapy at home, your oxygen provider will be contacted by the hospital. They will be told how much oxygen you need and the flow rate of oxygen required. Your oxygen provider will then arrange for the oxygen equipment and subsequent re-supplies to be delivered to your home.

Long-term oxygen therapy

Long-term oxygen therapy is usually prescribed for people who require oxygen frequently on a daily basis. It has been shown that you will need to be receiving oxygen for at least 15 hours a day in order to derive benefit from long-term oxygen therapy.

Long-term oxygen therapy may increase life expectancy. It can also help improve alertness, breathlessness, fatigue and sleep. You cannot become addicted to oxygen as you can with certain drugs. Oxygen sustains life and it may help improve your symptoms and allow you to live life to the fullest.

COPD is a progressive condition and once you are receiving long-term oxygen therapy it is likely that you will continue to use it for the rest of your life as your need for oxygen increases with time.

It will, however, have a significant impact on your lifestyle. Activities of daily living will have to be adjusted accordingly in order to accommodate and to ensure adequate oxygen therapy. Most people will keep the oxygen on overnight while sleeping to allow for more free time without oxygen during the day in order to make up the 15 hours a day that is required.

Oxygen concentrator

An oxygen concentrator is used to deliver continuous oxygen. It uses room air to concentrate oxygen and runs on electricity. You will be given either a mask or a tube, known as a nasal cannula, that has two small prongs that fit into your nostrils to use with the oxygen.

It is important that you keep your oxygen concentrator in a well-ventilated area because it requires good clean air to operate properly. You should also ensure that your oxygen concentrator is serviced regularly so that it continues to work properly. You should receive instructions from your oxygen provider about this.

Once you are started on long-term oxygen therapy, you will be seen at least once a year in the hospital chest clinic. This is to assess how you are getting on with the oxygen therapy. It will also provide you with an opportunity to raise any questions that you may have.

Short-burst oxygen therapy

You may find that you have been prescribed oxygen to be used occasionally rather than continuously. This is to help during moments when you may feel more breathless than usual. This can be at times when you are resting or during periods just before and after physical activity.

Short-burst oxygen therapy is usually used for about 10 to 20 minutes at a time to relieve breathlessness. It is often delivered from an oxygen cylinder at home. A typical oxygen cylinder usually provides oxygen for up to 11 hours using a flow rate of 2 litres a minute.

It is important that you keep the oxygen cylinder away from any heat source such as cookers or open

Oxygen concentrator

Electricity powers a compressor that forces room air through chemical filters, which remove much of the nitrogen from the air – leaving an oxygen-rich gas.

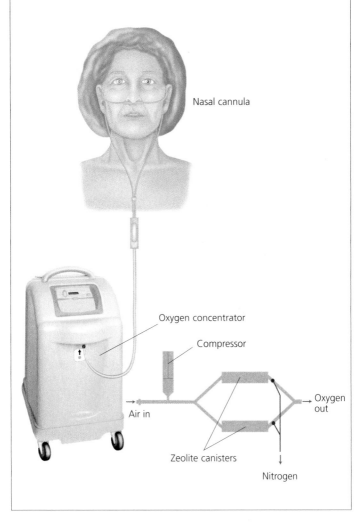

Nasal cannula

Oxygen concentrator

Compressor

Air in

Oxygen out

Nitrogen

Zeolite canisters

Oxygen cylinder

Cylinders contain compressed gaseous oxygen. Cylinders are refilled by a gas supplier.

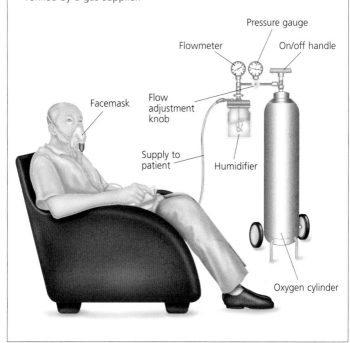

fires. Heat will cause a build-up of pressure. This may result in rupture of the oxygen cylinder should the pressure relief device fail to function.

Ambulatory oxygen therapy

Ambulatory oxygen therapy is prescribed for people who are mobile and who are able to leave the house. It is used during physical activity associated with daily living. It can also be given to people who are already receiving long-term oxygen therapy.

Portable oxygen

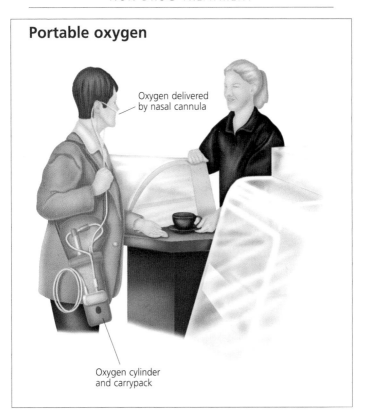

Oxygen delivered by nasal cannula

Oxygen cylinder and carrypack

Ambulatory oxygen therapy is delivered from portable devices that can be carried over the shoulder or as a backpack using special carriers. They enable greater freedom and the ability to engage in more activities. Portable oxygen cylinders are available. However, because they are generally smaller than home oxygen cylinders, they typically last for only up to two hours using flow rates of two litres a minute.

Oxygen in compressed and cooled liquid form provides the best portability and lasts longer than conventional portable oxygen cylinders. Liquid oxygen is transformed into gas through a warming process before use. There is usually enough liquid oxygen in a portable container to last for about eight hours at a flow rate of two litres a minute.

You should not feel ashamed when using oxygen outdoors. Most people are understanding and will see that you are leading your life to the best of your ability. Be confident and do not let this minor inconvenience stop you from staying active.

Travel and oxygen therapy

You should be able to travel regardless of whether or not you are currently receiving oxygen therapy. However, you should always see your doctor first to ensure that it is safe to do so. This is especially important if you are planning a journey on an aeroplane.

Your doctor will get an idea of the level of oxygen in your blood by using a simple probe that usually rests on the tip of one of your fingers, which connects to an oxygen saturation monitor. This is known as pulse oximetry. If the oxygen level is too low, your doctor will refer you to a chest specialist.

You will then be assessed in hospital to see whether you will require some supplemental oxygen during your flight. This evaluation of fitness to fly will usually involve measuring the response of your body to a simulated aircraft cabin environment.

Should you require in-flight oxygen, you will need to contact the airline with which you are flying to let them know. The airline will then contact the hospital to ask for information about how much oxygen is required and at what flow rate it is to be delivered. Please be aware

Pulse oximetry

Your doctor can quickly assess the level of oxygen in your blood using a probe that clips on your fingertip. A light beam is used to assess the oxygen level so the procedure is entirely painless.

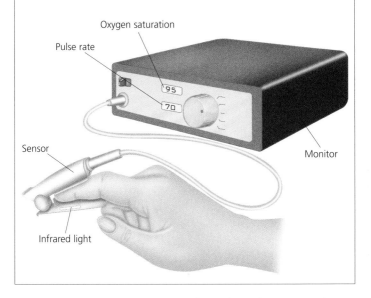

Oxygen saturation

Pulse rate

95

70

Sensor

Monitor

Infrared light

that there is usually a charge from the airline to supply the oxygen. This is in addition to your normal ticket fare.

On some occasions, there will be people whose oxygen levels are too low to allow safe flying, even with supplemental oxygen, whereas, in others, oxygen therapy may not be suitable. Do not be discouraged if you are told that you cannot fly. Think of other alternatives such as a journey by either land or sea.

Careful planning will be required when travelling, especially if you are currently on oxygen therapy. You will need to arrange for oxygen to be used during your journey and also for oxygen to be provided at your destination. It will be difficult but not impossible.

Find out from friends who may have been in a similar situation and how they managed. See your doctor who may be able to provide help or useful advice.

Artificial ventilation

Despite being on all possible treatment during a flare-up in hospital, you may find yourself still very breathless. The hospital doctor may decide to put you on a breathing machine if you continue to struggle.

The machine known as a ventilator will help with the work of breathing. They generally work by generating a positive pressure to help deliver air into your lungs. It is particularly useful if you are beginning to tire as a result of exhaustion.

Ventilation is broadly divided into invasive and non-invasive.

Invasive ventilation

Invasive ventilation involves general anaesthesia and a tube being inserted into the trachea (windpipe) known as an intubation. The tube is connected to the ventilator machine, which helps you breathe. You will be required to stay in an intensive care unit while you are receiving this form of treatment. You will also remain sedated throughout until you are well enough for the tube to be removed, known as an extubation.

Non-invasive ventilation

Non-invasive ventilation is generally preferred as no sedation or intubation is involved. You will, however, be required to use a mask that is securely fastened to prevent air from leaking out. It will be uncomfortable at first but do not worry. As you get used to the mask and to the pressure generated by the ventilator, you

Invasive ventilation

The patient is first anaesthetised. The doctor uses a laryngoscope to see down the throat. The endotracheal tube (ETT) is passed into the trachea (windpipe). The cuff of the ETT is inflated to create a seal within the trachea. The patient is then attached to the ventilator.

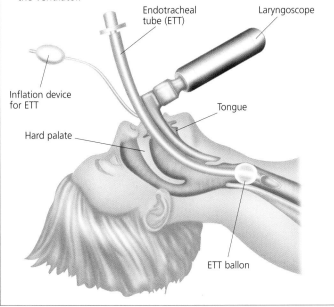

Endotracheal tube (ETT)

Laryngoscope

Inflation device for ETT

Tongue

Hard palate

ETT ballon

will find that your breathing will start to get easier. Non-invasive ventilation can be performed in a specially monitored unit within a hospital ward.

You will gradually be weaned from the ventilator the moment you start to recover. Once again, as at the start of ventilation, it may be uncomfortable. You may find that you need to breathe harder without the ventilator. This is normal and is to be expected. Remember, while you were on the ventilator, it was helping you with the work of breathing. Without it, you are doing all the work by yourself again.

Non-invasive ventilation

This is primarily aimed at minimising patient discomfort and the complications associated with invasive ventilation.

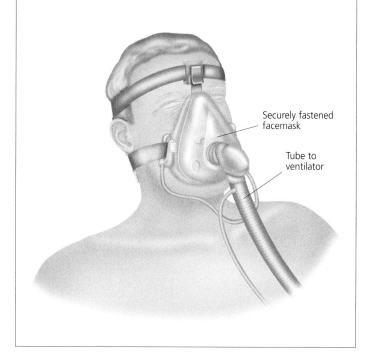

Securely fastened facemask

Tube to ventilator

Surgery

Surgery for COPD is a difficult operation with many potential complications. Some people who have the operation do not survive it. Most people with COPD will not be offered surgery because many will not benefit from it. For the few who may gain benefit, strict selection criteria are used. This is to ensure optimal outcome with the best chance of survival.

Lung volume reduction surgery

The most common surgical procedure is known as lung volume reduction surgery (LVRS). It involves removing parts of the lung that are damaged in COPD. This will allow other parts of the lung that are healthy to work better where the effort of breathing can now be concentrated upon. There should be an improvement in breathing after successful surgery because LVRS will also allow the diaphragm to return to its normal shape, enabling more efficient breathing.

Bullectomy

There is also another form of surgery known as bullectomy. This type of surgery is suitable only for people who have a large bulla. A bulla is a ball-shaped air sac that has formed as a result of air trapping in a damaged part of the lung. Breathing should improve as the healthier lungs start to work better after removal of the bulla.

Lung transplantation

People with COPD may also be considered for lung transplantation. The selection process is rigorous and there are many strict criteria to be followed. If you are found to be suitable for lung transplantation, you will be put on a waiting list. Time will be needed to find a matching donor. There is also a shortage of donor organs nationally.

Lung volume reduction surgery (LVRS)

This is a surgical procedure performed to remove diseased, emphysematous lung tissue. This procedure:

- reduces the size of an over-inflated lung
- allows the expansion of the remaining, often more functional lung.

The lungs are made up of lobes as shown below.

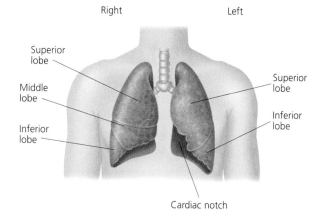

Front view of healthy lungs

Right | Left

Superior lobe
Middle lobe
Inferior lobe

Superior lobe
Inferior lobe

Cardiac notch

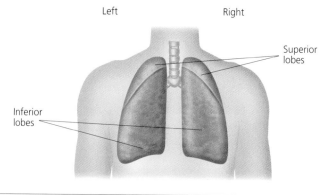

Back view of healthy lungs

Left | Right

Superior lobes

Inferior lobes

KEY POINTS

- Oxygen therapy may be required in some but not all people with COPD; there are strict selection criteria to be followed before oxygen therapy can be prescribed

- You and others around you must not smoke if you are receiving oxygen therapy; it is dangerous and can result in severe burns and even death, and you will not be offered home oxygen therapy if you are currently smoking

- Should you require oxygen therapy, your doctor will decide on whether you will need to use it only occasionally or regularly for a minimum of at least 15 hours a day

- You will need to see your doctor before embarking on a journey that involves air travel

- Surgery is suitable only for a highly selected group of people with COPD; major lung surgery is difficult and complications may be fatal

Support for COPD patients

Stopping smoking

Smoking is now recognised as the most important source of preventable sickness and premature death worldwide. Smoking causes addiction, anxiety, asthma, bladder cancer, blindness, cervical cancer, COPD, cot death, dementia, diabetes, heart attack, heart disease, impotency, infertility, kidney cancer, laryngeal (voicebox) cancer, leukaemia, lip cancer, low birth weight, lung cancer, miscarriage, mouth cancer, oesophageal (gullet) cancer, pancreatic cancer, pneumonia, poor blood circulation, poor wound healing, premature birth, stomach cancer, stomach ulcer, stress, stroke, throat cancer and many other diseases.

It does not matter if you have been a smoker for many years. It is never too late to stop. The immediate benefits of stopping smoking are immense, even if you have smoked for more than 20 years. Within half an hour of stopping smoking, your blood pressure and heart rate will improve while your hands and feet start to warm up. The oxygen level in your blood will rise within 8 hours and your risk of having a heart attack will reduce within 24 hours.

Your smell and taste improve within 48 hours while your breathing becomes easier within 72 hours and your blood circulation improves within 2 weeks. Within a month, your lung function will increase by a third and, within 3 months, physical activity will be significantly easier as your blood circulation and lung function continues to improve.

You will feel considerably less breathless as coughing, congestion and fatigue lessen within 9 months. Your risk of suffering from heart disease will be halved within a year and your chances of having a stroke will be reduced to that of a person who has never smoked within 5 years. You will have halved the risk of developing lung cancer within 10 years, and reduced the risk of having heart disease and premature death to a level similar to that of a life-long non-smoker within 15 years. There are, therefore, many great benefits to be had not only by stopping smoking immediately but also by maintaining total abstinence from tobacco smoke.

Giving up smoking is not easy. Nicotine, which is one of the chemicals present in tobacco smoke, is highly addictive. Smokers become dependent on nicotine. Once absorbed into the bloodstream, nicotine is as addictive as cocaine or heroin.

The first step in giving up smoking is making the decision to stop smoking. Once the decision is made, the second step is to have the determination to stop.

Smoking may be like an old habit that is difficult but not impossible to break. Try to get your mind off smoking when temptation beckons. Engage in different leisure activities or start a new hobby.

You may experience lapses when your willpower fails you. It does not matter as long as you pick yourself up again. Stay true to your decision and continue with your determination to stop smoking. You can succeed.

Remember that you are not alone in your struggle. There are many people who have been in your position and have successfully given up smoking. Your doctor will be able to offer help and support in addition to referring you to your local NHS Stop Smoking Service, which usually comprises doctors, nurses, pharmacists and specialist advisers.

You are also more likely to succeed in giving up smoking if others around you do not smoke. If there are members of your family who smoke, they can help you greatly by stopping smoking themselves at the same time.

Nicotine replacement

You may feel an unbearable craving or become very irritable when you first give up smoking. These are called withdrawal symptoms, and they are caused by addiction to nicotine and can be expected. A way of helping with withdrawal symptoms is to use nicotine replacement therapies. Your doctor or pharmacist will be able to advise you further on this.

Using nicotine products may increase your success in giving up smoking. They come in many different forms. The most popular are nicotine patches that you can stick on your skin, usually on your arm. A patch will typically last for one day. These patches contain nicotine that is released slowly into your body, helping you with your craving and withdrawal.

Your doctor will be able to give you an initial prescription of at least a week's supply, which can then

Nicotine patch mode of action

Nicotine replacement therapies can help you with withdrawal symptoms. Ask your doctor or pharmacist about this.

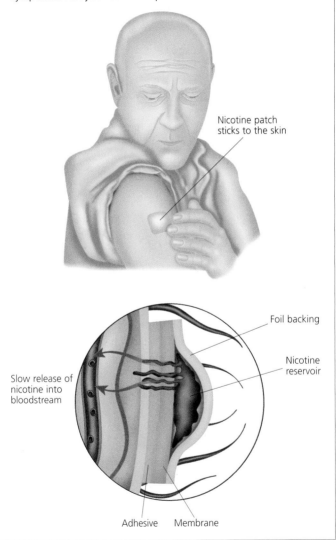

Nicotine patch sticks to the skin

Foil backing

Nicotine reservoir

Slow release of nicotine into bloodstream

Adhesive   Membrane

be extended to another three weeks depending on your progress. Sometimes it may be necessary to extend the treatment period further.

You will have to work closely with your doctor, who may also refer you to a smoking adviser in order to help you tackle your withdrawal symptoms and cravings in a structured manner.

Nicotine products are also available as chewing gums, tablets or even lozenges. Sometimes they can also be found as nasal sprays and inhalator devices. Choose the nicotine replacement therapy that suits you best and helps you most in your battle to stay off smoking.

Non-nicotine medication
Bupropion (Zyban)
This is a non-nicotine medication that may help when you are ready and motivated to stop smoking. It breaks the cycle of nicotine addiction by working directly on the addiction and withdrawal pathways in the brain. It affects the urge to keep on smoking and reduces the cravings for cigarettes.

It can also help with withdrawal symptoms as your body adjusts to being without nicotine. It may cause dry mouth, headaches, sleep disturbances and, rarely, seizures. See your doctor who will be able to offer you more advice on this medication.

Typically you would decide on a date that you would stop smoking. You would then start treatment while you are still smoking two weeks before that quit date in order for it to start working. Your desire to smoke will gradually lessen as the treatment begins to work. The duration of treatment is usually for eight weeks on average.

Varenicline (Champix)

This medication may help you quit smoking by reducing your craving and your sense of pleasure from smoking. It is non-nicotine based and acts by blocking out the effects of nicotine in the brain. It reduces the feeling of satisfaction that you get from smoking. It may also cause nausea.

Treatment is commenced two weeks before your quit date and usually lasts for about 12 weeks.

Cut down or stop?

It is generally felt that the best way to stop smoking is the outright stop approach with appropriate support. The cut down first and then stop approach should be reserved only for smokers who would otherwise not consider stopping at all.

Pulmonary rehabilitation

Pulmonary rehabilitation is an individually tailored course or programme aimed at helping you cope better with COPD. Health professionals from various specialities endeavour to provide help and support you throughout the programme. This is known as a multidisciplinary team approach.

Pulmonary rehabilitation courses are held in many different places ranging from a department in your local hospital to a village hall in your local community. It will depend very much on the area where you live as well as the local availability of staff and equipment. You will have to be referred by the chest specialist in order to be enrolled on a pulmonary rehabilitation course. It is also likely that you will be placed on a waiting list because places on these popular courses are often limited.

Physiotherapists

Physiotherapists will teach you how to strengthen your muscles through exercises tailored to suit you. The purpose of these exercises is to increase the strength and capacity for work of your muscles.

These exercises generally target the entire body although some emphasis may be placed on certain muscle groups. For example, you may find that, by improving the muscles in your chest, you are able to breathe better.

Through following a routine and graded exercise programme, you may become stronger and able to do things with less effort than before. For instance, you may find that you are able to climb stairs without getting too breathless or you may be able to walk further without having to rest so often. The improvement gained in your breathing may be as good as that obtained from your inhaler therapy.

Specialist nurses

Specialist nurses will be able to provide you with the latest developments in managing COPD. They will be able to teach you more about the condition and give you important information.

You will learn how to cope better and be taught what to do in the event of a flare-up. Your inhaler technique and device will also be assessed. This is to make sure that your current inhaler device suits you and that you are able to use it properly.

Occupational therapists

Occupational therapists will be able to offer advice on how to manage the physical difficulties that you may be experiencing with COPD. They will provide useful suggestions about how to modify your home or workplace to make it more comfortable for you.

You may find that you require help with climbing stairs or help with getting in and out of the bath. Occupational therapists will be able to assess your needs and possibly provide you with equipment such as a stair lift. They may also suggest useful alterations or adaptations in your home.

Dietitians

Dietitians will teach you about diet and healthy eating. It is important that you eat well in order to maintain your weight. Weight loss is usually a feature of severe COPD. Dietitians will be able to address this and provide expert help.

Healthy eating will also improve your general well-being and resistance to illness. You will be shown the best types of food to eat. You will also be advised to avoid foods that are unhealthy.

Home-support schemes

You may find that, after being in hospital for a flare-up, you are discharged home early. Sometimes, after careful assessment, a hospital doctor sends you home on the very same day that you go in. This is to minimise the risk of getting an infection from hospital. Once at home, specialist nurses will support you and visit you daily. These schemes are known as hospital-at-home or assisted-discharge schemes.

Specialist nurses will provide you with equipment that you may need such as a nebuliser during your flare-up. They will check on your treatment and ensure that you are improving. Many people with flare-ups who are discharged on a home-support scheme do well.

If, however, you are not getting better or are getting worse at any stage during your treatment at home, you will be advised to return to hospital immediately. Specialist nurses will then arrange for you to be admitted directly to a medical ward where you will receive further treatment.

Immunisation

To reduce the risk of a flare-up, it is recommended that you receive protection against flu. See your doctor to receive your yearly immunisation, which is usually given during the winter months.

The flu vaccine is made up of killed or inactivated flu virus. This is necessary in order to stimulate your immune system to combat the real-life flu virus if and when your body encounters it.

Side effects

Some people may experience soreness, redness and swelling at the site of injection after the flu immunisation. These symptoms should usually settle. If it does not get better or the injection site gets worse, you must see your doctor.

Besides the local effects of the flu immunisation on the injection site, you may also experience some side effects that affect your body in general. It is very rare that this happens. However, you may get aches and pains in your body after the immunisation. It is usually more common in people who have been immunised for the first time.

You may also develop a fever after flu immunisation. Simple medication such as paracetamol may provide relief for your general aches and pains, as well as help reduce any high temperatures.

With each subsequent immunisation, you should experience fewer of these side effects.

Can anyone be immunised?

It is important to realise that not everyone may be suitable to receive the flu immunisation. This is true if you are allergic to eggs because they are used to make the vaccine. Please see your doctor about this. Also, further immunisation may not be advisable if you had a bad reaction to the previous one. Once again, your doctor will be able to offer advice on this.

Having the flu vaccine does not guarantee that you will not catch flu. Some people have been known to catch flu even after having the immunisation. This is rather rare and the flu is usually much milder compared with flu in someone who has not been immunised. It is also important to realise that having the flu vaccine will not protect you against other viruses, including the common cold.

Why do I need annual immunisation?

The flu vaccine is given every year for several reasons. The flu viruses causing flu in one year may be different in the next year. This is because there are many different strains of the viruses around and the strains responsible for flu tend to vary from year to year. Therefore, a flu vaccine this year may not be effective the next year when a different strain of flu virus emerges.

Also the protection offered by the flu vaccine tends to diminish over a period of one year. For these reasons, you should keep your annual appointment for your yearly flu immunisation.

In addition, you are also encouraged to receive immunisation against the pneumococcal bacteria that commonly cause pneumonia. Most people will require the vaccine once only. See your doctor for advice.

Avoiding infections

It may also be useful to avoid crowded places especially during the winter months. When there are a lot of people in a confined place, there is always an increased risk of catching an infection.

Many infections such as flu and pneumonia are spread through the air by infectious droplets, usually generated by coughing. It may be best to turn away or politely walk away if someone near you is unwell and coughing.

They will understand about your vulnerability to developing infections and the necessary precautions that are required to minimise them. Remember, if your friend or relative is unwell with flu or pneumonia, it will be advisable to visit them only after they have made a complete recovery.

You can always show your concern by talking to them over the phone or by sending them a 'get well soon' card. You may even wish to communicate by email to convey your messages.

If you have people caring for you at home, the single most important precaution that you can take to prevent infections is to ask your carers always to wash their hands before and after attending to you.

Use plenty of liquid soap and warm water. The hands should be scrubbed for at least 20 seconds. Do not forget the fingernails either. Proper hand washing will minimise your risk of getting infections from contaminated hands.

You should also keep your inhaler, spacer and nebuliser devices clean at all times. This will not only help to ensure that they continue to function properly but also aid in minimising infections.

If you use oxygen devices, it is important that you clean the air filter and compressor filter regularly, in accordance with the manufacturers' instructions, to prevent contamination and infection.

Lung cancer

There is an increased risk of developing lung cancer with a previous history of smoking. Lung cancer is uncontrolled growth of abnormal cells in lung tissue.

The chance of having lung cancer is further increased if you are still smoking. It is important to be aware of certain warning signs that may indicate lung cancer and see your doctor if:

- you start coughing up blood

- you become excessively tired

- you have a poor appetite or start to lose weight without any obvious reasons.

Please note, however, that having these symptoms does not necessarily mean that you have lung cancer. You will require further investigations and may be referred to a chest specialist in the hospital.

Outlook for COPD patients

The damage to the lungs in COPD is irreversible. However, progression of the condition may be slowed down. Breathlessness may also be improved. This can be achieved by learning as much as you can about your condition and how best to manage it.

Abundant information is available through your GP surgery, hospital, local support groups, media, books and the internet.

With the correct treatment and support, you will be able to improve your quality of life and cope better with your breathlessness.

You will also be able to recognise when to seek help from your doctor and learn how to minimise a flare-up. Never be disheartened and always remain positive.

KEY POINTS

■ Stopping smoking is a very important first step in battling COPD; support is available to help you stop smoking if you are struggling

■ Learning more about COPD will help you cope better with the condition

■ Attending pulmonary rehabilitation is a good way to improve your quality of life

■ Home support schemes are becoming very popular and it is very likely that your local hospital will have such a scheme in place; it will help support you better at home while avoiding unnecessary prolonged stays in hospital

■ It is very important that you are up to date with your immunisations, so that flare-ups can be kept to a minimum

■ Try to maintain a positive outlook on life

Living with COPD

Exercise

Any form of exercise will be useful. It does not necessarily have to involve going to your local gymnasium. Gentle exercise such as brisk walking or even a stroll in the park will help keep you active.

There will always be some people who will be able to do more than others. It is important that you do not get carried away and over-exert yourself. Know your limitations and do not exceed them.

Some people with COPD may be receiving home oxygen therapy. You should not be confined to your home as a result of this. See your doctor to discuss portable oxygen devices that you can easily carry with you when leaving home.

Always try to stay physically active. It will improve your blood circulation and help get much needed oxygen throughout your body. You will feel better for it. You may find that you are unable to do much at the beginning but your stamina will improve with time. It will be a gradual process. Continue to stay focused and committed.

Your physiotherapist will be able to advise you on the appropriate exercises to undertake. There are various different types of exercises available. Some are general and will exercise different areas of your body. Others are more specialised and will focus on developing a specific area such as the upper body and chest to help with your breathing.

COPD management techniques

You may find the following information provided by the US Cleveland Clinic Foundation helpful. They provide practical and useful advice on controlled coughing, diaphragmatic breathing and pursed-lip breathing.

Controlled coughing

COPD can cause your lungs to produce excess mucus, leading to frequent coughing. Not all coughs are effective in clearing excess mucus from the lungs. Explosive or uncontrolled coughing causes airways to collapse and spasm, trapping mucus.

The effective, or controlled, cough comes from deep within the lungs and has just enough force to loosen and carry mucus through the airways without causing them to narrow and collapse. Controlled coughing saves energy and, therefore, oxygen.

Controlled coughing technique

To cough effectively:

- Sit on a chair or on the edge of your bed, with both feet on the floor. Lean slightly forward. Relax.

- Fold your arms across your abdomen and breathe in slowly through your nose. The power of the cough comes from moving air.

- To exhale: lean forward, pressing your arms against your abdomen. Cough two to three times through a slightly open mouth. Coughs should be short and sharp. The first cough loosens the mucus and moves it through the airways. The second and third coughs enable you to cough the mucus up and out.

- Breathe in again by 'sniffing' slowly and gently through your nose. This gentle breath helps prevent mucus from moving back down your airways.

- Rest.

- Perform again if needed.

Tips

Avoid breathing in quickly and deeply through your mouth after coughing. Quick breaths can interfere with the movement of mucus up and out of the lungs and can cause uncontrolled coughing.

Drink six to eight glasses of fluid per day unless your doctor has told you to limit your fluid intake. When mucus is thin, coughing is easier.

Use the controlled coughing technique after you use your bronchodilator medication or any time that you feel congested with mucus.

Mucus-clearing devices

If you have trouble coughing up secretions, your doctor may prescribe a mucus-clearing device, such as the flutter device or the positive expiratory pressure (PEP) valve. There are other mucus-clearing devices on the market that may be prescribed by your doctor.

Flutter device

A mucus-clearing device such as the flutter helps

loosen mucus in the airways so that you can cough it up more easily. The flutter consists of:

- a mouthpiece

- protective cover

- high-density stainless steel ball

- a circular cone.

When you exhale, your breath moves the steel ball inside, causing vibrations in your lungs. These vibrations loosen the mucus so that it can move up and out of the airways.

Positive expiratory pressure valve

The PEP valve generates resistance to the air that you breathe out, called positive expiratory pressure. The resistance from the PEP can be varied. The setting that should work best for you is determined by your doctor or therapist.

To use the PEP valve, place the mouthpiece in your mouth, seal your lips around it, take a deep breath using your diaphragm and breathe out slowly with a moderate force through the one-way valve for as long as you can.

The increased pressure in the airways will give you the feeling to cough. When you feel the urge to cough, take a deep breath in, hold for one to three seconds, and cough to loosen the mucus.

Diaphragmatic breathing

The diaphragm is the most efficient muscle of breathing. It is a large, dome-shaped muscle located at the base of the lungs. Your abdominal muscles help move the diaphragm and give you more power to empty your

Flutter device

This is a mucus-clearing device. The oscillation of the steel ball sets up a 'fluttering' back pressure in the lungs, which can loosen mucus – so it can move out of the airways.

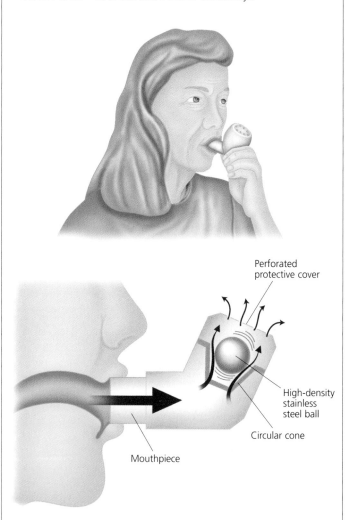

Perforated protective cover

High-density stainless steel ball

Circular cone

Mouthpiece

Positive expiratory pressure (PEP) valve

A mask covers your mouth and nose. A valve in the mask generates a variable resistance to your exhaled breath. The increased pressure in your airways will make you want to cough – which will loosen mucus.

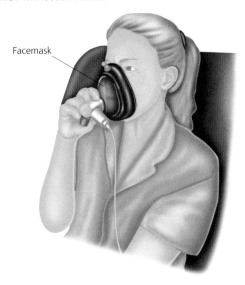

Facemask

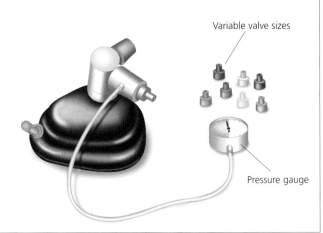

Variable valve sizes

Pressure gauge

lungs. However, COPD may prevent the diaphragm from working effectively.

When you have lung disease, such as COPD, air often becomes trapped in the lungs, pushing down on the diaphragm. The neck and chest muscles must then assume an increased share of the work of breathing. This can leave the diaphragm weakened and flattened, causing it to work less efficiently.

Diaphragmatic breathing is intended to help you use the diaphragm correctly while breathing to:

- strengthen the diaphragm

- decrease the work input into breathing by slowing your breathing rate

- decrease oxygen demand.

Diaphragmatic breathing technique

1 Lie on your back on a flat surface or in bed, with your knees bent and your head supported. You can use a pillow under your knees to support your legs. Place one hand on your upper chest and the other just below your rib cage. This will allow you to feel your diaphragm move as you breathe.

2 Breathe in slowly through your nose so that your stomach moves out against your hand. The hand on your chest should remain as still as possible.

3 Tighten your stomach muscles, letting them fall inward as you exhale through pursed lips. The hand on your upper chest must remain as still as possible.

When you first learn the diaphragmatic breathing technique, it may be easier for you to follow the instructions lying down, as described above. As you gain more practice, you can try the diaphragmatic breathing technique while sitting in a chair, as described below.

To perform this exercise while sitting in a chair:

1 Sit comfortably, with your knees bent and your shoulders, head and neck relaxed.

2 Place one hand on your upper chest and the other just below your ribcage. This will allow you to feel your diaphragm move as you breathe.

3 Tighten your stomach muscles, letting them fall inward as you exhale through pursed lips. The hand on your upper chest must remain as still as possible.

Note: you may notice that an increased effort will be needed to use the diaphragm correctly. At first, you will probably get tired while doing this exercise. But keep at it, because, with continued practice, diaphragmatic breathing will become easy and automatic.

How often should I practise this exercise?
At first, practise this exercise for 5 to 10 minutes about three to four times per day. Gradually increase the amount of time that you spend doing this exercise, and perhaps even increase the effort of the exercise if you are doing it lying down by placing a book on your abdomen.

Pursed-lip breathing
Pursed-lip breathing is one of the simplest ways to control shortness of breath. It provides a quick and easy way to slow your pace of breathing, making each breath more effective.

What does pursed-lip breathing do?

Pursed-lip breathing:

- improves ventilation

- releases trapped air in the lungs

- keeps the airways open longer and decreases the work of breathing

- prolongs exhalation to slow the breathing rate

- improves breathing patterns by moving old air out of the lungs and allowing new air to enter the lungs

- relieves shortness of breath

- causes general relaxation.

When should I use this technique?

Use this technique during the difficult part of any activity, such as bending, lifting or stair climbing.

Practise this technique four or five times a day at first so that you can get the correct breathing pattern. The technique is as follows:

1 Relax your neck and shoulder muscles.

2 Breathe in or inhale slowly through your nose for two counts, keeping your mouth closed. Do not take a deep breath – a normal breath will do. It may help to count to yourself: inhale, one, two.

3 Pucker or 'purse' your lips as if you were going to whistle or gently flicker the flame of a candle.

4 Breathe out or exhale slowly and gently through your pursed lips while counting to four. It may help to count to yourself: exhale, one, two, three, four.

With regular practice, this technique will seem natural to you.

Diet

It is important that you maintain a healthy diet. Many people with COPD commonly find that they have a poor appetite. This inadvertently leads to a poor eating habit, resulting in weight loss. You need to try your best to avoid being undernourished and underweight because staying healthy and strong will help improve your breathing.

You must ensure that you maintain an adequate intake of food and fluids, even if you do not feel like it

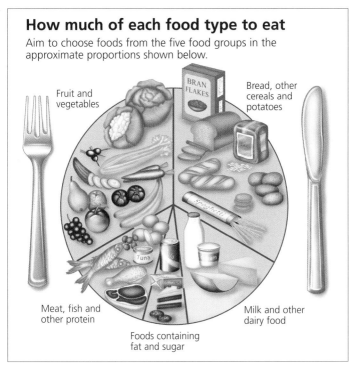

How much of each food type to eat

Aim to choose foods from the five food groups in the approximate proportions shown below.

Fruit and vegetables

Bread, other cereals and potatoes

Meat, fish and other protein

Milk and other dairy food

Foods containing fat and sugar

at times. Eating regularly and properly will help you get the correct amount of essential minerals and vitamins that your body requires.

You will also need sufficient protein in your diet to help maintain your muscles and calcium to keep your bones healthy.

An adequate amount of fibre available from fruit and vegetables is also important to maintain regular bowel motion and general health.

Your doctor will be able to refer you to a dietitian who can advise you with regard to good eating habits.

Depression

You may occasionally feel down as a result of the limitations that come along with your COPD. You may find that you can no longer do the things that you used to do or enjoyed doing. You may find that you have to make compromises in your life. You may ask yourself what is the point of going on in life if it is so constricted and limited.

It is important to appreciate that what you are going through mentally is normal and is to be expected. This is especially true when you have to live with a chronic disabling condition such as COPD. However, you must be quick to recognise the symptoms of depression and take appropriate action before it gets hold of you.

Look out for symptoms such as lack of energy and excessive tiredness, no longer enjoying the things that used to make you happy, feeling sad and miserable all the time, waking up in the early hours of the morning and not being able to sleep again, or simply just not being bothered to get up out of bed for fear of facing the day ahead.

You must not leave depression unaddressed. A vicious cycle may develop and spiral you into deeper depression. It may then be difficult to get out of the feeling of constant despair. Recognise the symptoms early and seek help.

See your doctor who will be sympathetic and understand what you are going through. Your doctor may also give you information about joining support groups that will put you in touch with other people who are in a similar situation as yourself. Talk to your friends or relatives. Do not try to deal with depression on your own.

Daily activity
It is likely that you may have to make some adjustments to certain aspects of your daily living.

Climbing stairs
Some people with COPD may find it difficult to climb stairs because they get too breathless. Some would struggle and have to stop in the middle of the flight of stairs. Others would not even attempt it for fear of starting a flare-up.

There are a few things you may try to improve the situation. If you are able to get to the top of the stairs without stopping but find that you are breathless after, you can try to use your reliever medication before climbing the stairs. This may help ease your breathlessness once you get to the top. If you are still breathless, do not hesitate to take more of your reliever medication.

Stair lifts and elevators may also help in getting you upstairs. See your doctor to discuss what is available for you. Arranging for a stair lift or elevator will usually involve key health workers such as occupational therapists and social workers.

Some people with COPD find that they do not wish to go upstairs anymore even with help from stair lifts or elevators. In such instances, the downstairs floor can be converted to include bedrooms and bathrooms, so that daily living would be convenient without having to go upstairs.

There may also be occasions when renovations cannot be physically carried out in your current home. In such instances, you may be advised to move to a more convenient home such as a bungalow. Your key health worker will be able to offer advice and guidance.

Leaving the house

COPD may affect you in such a way that it is no longer easy for you to do your daily shopping without getting too breathless. Your doctor may be able to help you by suggesting and arranging for a carer to visit you.

Your carer may help fully with your shopping without you having to leave the house. However, it is best to try to stay as active as possible. Use every opportunity you can to venture out of the house, even if it is just to the front gate.

If you like going out shopping, your carer may provide transportation, or may help in packing and carrying your shopping. You may also wish to consider using a scooter or a wheelchair to help you move around. Your doctor will be able to provide you with more information about getting these arranged.

Meal times

Cooking your daily meal may become difficult. If this is the case, a carer may be able to help cook your meals for you. Your carer may also be able to wash and clean up after as well. If there are no carers available, your health worker may suggest that you get your meals delivered to you using the community meals service that is available in your area.

Hygiene

It is important that personal hygiene is maintained at all times. If you find that you can no longer do any housework because of the limitations imposed on you by COPD, then you must seek advice from your doctor. Your health worker may arrange for carers to visit you once a day or even a few times a day depending on you requirements. Your carer will be able to help with daily chores and housework such as cleaning, cooking, emptying the rubbish and general tidying up around the house.

Some adjustments may have to be made to your bathroom. Your doctor will usually refer you to the occupational therapists who will visit you at home to look at the practical difficulties that you may have and work with you to identify your needs. Hand and grab rails may be installed to help you get in and out of the bath. A stool and grab rail may allow you to shower sitting down. It may be useful to have a hand-held telephone within easy reach just in case of emergencies while in the bathroom.

Some people may find that the steam generated from hot showers affects their breathing. You can help minimise this by leaving the bathroom door or window slightly ajar. If your shower has a glass door, then leave this slightly open so that steam can escape.

Fresh air

Air that is free from pollutants and irritants is desirable. Unfortunately, in the world we live in today, it is not always easy to attain such purity in the air we breathe. Therefore, it is important to try to minimise any exposure that may worsen your COPD.

Try to avoid breathing in fumes from paints and solvents. They can trigger a flare-up. Also some people find that perfumes make their breathing worse. Try to keep your home well ventilated at all times. When cooking, always ensure that the extractor fan is on. It would also be preferable to close the kitchen door directly leading to your living room or any other room but leave the windows in your kitchen open. This is to prevent any smoke or mist from cooking spreading around the house because they may worsen your breathing.

It is usually best if you can try to go out for walks as much as possible when the weather is good. This will allow you to get some gentle exercise.

However, air that is too cold may make breathing worse in some people with COPD. Caution is therefore required, especially when there are strong winds that will make walking harder or when the weather is cold.

Hopefully by now you will have stopped smoking. It will also be necessary for you to make sure that no one around you smokes. Passive smoking may cause the same health problems as active smoking. It is best that you avoid places where people are likely to smoke. No matter how well a smoking area is ventilated, the air is always unhealthy because there is a lot of smoke constantly produced by smokers. Smoke usually lingers on for a considerable amount of time.

Avoid dusty places, for instance where construction is being carried out such as building sites. Also try to keep away from garages or congested roads where exhaust fumes are being constantly produced.

Both industrial building dust and motor exhaust fumes may make your breathing worse. If, however, going to these places is unavoidable, you should consider wearing an appropriate mask for protection. This should minimise your exposure to potentially harmful compounds.

Air pollution mask

The air that we breathe is not always as fresh as we would like. If you have to expose yourself to dust or other pollutants, use a mask for protection.

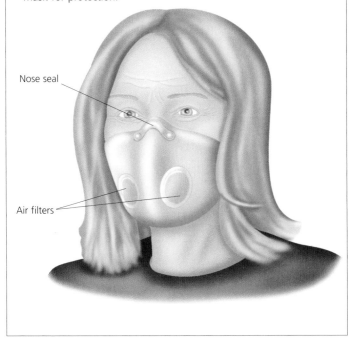

Nose seal

Air filters

KEY POINTS

- Try to remain as active as possible; physical activity no matter how little is important in keeping your body strong

- Know your limitations and do not exceed your boundaries

- Recognise depression early and seek help; never try to deal with depression on your own

- Maintain a healthy lifestyle and diet

Questions and answers

If COPD is irreversible, what is the point of giving up smoking?

Stopping smoking will stop the injury to your lungs caused by tobacco smoke. By removing the insult to your lungs, further damage is prevented. This will slow down the decline in your lung function. Most people derive immediate benefit as soon as they stop smoking. They feel that they can breathe better and are able to inhale deeper. Their sense of smell and taste also improves.

Remember, by stopping smoking, you will also reduce your risk of developing lung cancer and other medical problems such as heart disease and stroke.

People around you will benefit as well. Passive smoking causes chest problems in others and will also increase their risk of developing lung cancer.

You will also need to stop before you can be considered for home oxygen therapy should you require it to help you breathe better.

My grandfather smoked all his life but never had COPD. Why is this?

Most people who have been smoking for a long time have chronic bronchitis. However, only a sixth of them will go on to develop COPD.

The exact reason for this is not yet clear. Some people are more susceptible than others to the detrimental effects of tobacco smoke. This may be the result of individual differences in the way tobacco smoke is handled by our bodies.

My friend and I have similar breathing problems. Why has she been diagnosed with asthma and yet I have been told that I have COPD?

Although COPD and asthma can produce similar symptoms, they are very different conditions. The narrowing of the airways in COPD is predominantly irreversible. However, in asthma, the narrowed airways can be significantly widened by inhaler therapy leading to complete resolution of wheezing.

COPD is almost always associated with smoking. People who suffer from asthma, on the other hand, may be life-long non-smokers. People with COPD tend to cough and produce phlegm in the mornings. However, periodic wheezing especially during the nights may be more suggestive of asthma.

People with allergies are also more likely to develop asthma than COPD. Nevertheless, it is important to appreciate that there are some people who can suffer from both COPD and asthma.

There is blood in my phlegm. Should I be concerned?

You will need to see your doctor immediately. It is important that you provide your doctor with a detailed history including any recent weight loss, be it intentional or otherwise. Your doctor will need to examine you properly and you will be required to have a chest X-ray. This is to ensure that the cause of your coughing up blood is identified.

Unfortunately, people with COPD who have smoked have an increased risk of developing lung cancer. Coughing up blood may be one of the first signs that something is amiss. However, having blood in your phlegm does not necessarily mean that you have lung cancer. Other conditions such as a chest infection or pneumonia can result in similar symptoms.

I was admitted to hospital recently. Upon discharge, I was given different inhalers from the ones that I usually get from my local GP surgery. Now at home, I have so many different inhalers that I am getting confused as to which ones to use.

It is always important to clarify your medications with the nursing staff or doctor before leaving the hospital. The inhalers prescribed in hospital should replace your usual inhalers, which you were using before going into hospital. Therefore, you should stop your old inhalers and start using the new ones.

However, hospital doctors occasionally may not be aware of some of your usual inhalers. For that reason, if you are uncertain it is always best to consult your doctor to make sure that you are receiving the correct treatment. Take the discharge letter containing the medication details from the hospital with all your inhalers to your doctor who will then be able to help you.

I have been prescribed different medications and inhalers for my COPD. They do help with my breathlessness but why do they not take it away completely?

Therapy in COPD is generally aimed at improving symptoms such as breathlessness. They help to keep the airways open and reduce the amount of phlegm that is produced. During a flare-up, appropriate treatment can hasten recovery.

However, medications and inhalers prescribed for COPD do not repair the already damaged lung nor do they offer a cure. The narrowing of the airways found in COPD cannot be fully reversed with treatment. Therefore, a degree of residual breathlessness is to be expected even with maximum therapy.

Useful information

Where can I find out more?

We have included the following organisations because, on preliminary investigation, they may be of use to the reader. However, we do not have first-hand experience of each organisation and so cannot guarantee the organisation's integrity. The reader must therefore exercise his or her own discretion and judgement when making further enquiries.

General information

Benefits Enquiry Line

Tel: 0800 882200
Minicom: 0800 243355
Website: www.dwp.gov.uk
N. Ireland: 0800 220674

Government agency giving information and advice on sickness and disability benefits for people with disabilities and their carers.

British Lung Foundation
73–75 Goswell Road
London EC1V 7ER
Tel: 0845 850 5020
Website: www.lunguk.org

Only UK charity focusing on and tackling all aspects of more than 40 lung conditions, which, on average, affect one member of every family, from premature babies with breathing problems, to children with asthma and older people with lung cancer or COPD. Provides information and support while working to improve the quality of life of those living with a lung condition.

Cleveland Clinic Foundation
9500 Euclid Avenue
Cleveland, OH 44195
USA
Tel: +1 216 444 2200
Website: www.clevelandclinic.org

One of the world's largest and busiest health centres. Founded in 1921 as a not-for-profit group practice, integrating clinical and hospital care with physician education. Has an excellent department that is dedicated to providing patient education and health information.

Clinical Knowledge Summaries
Sowerby Centre for Health Informatics at Newcastle (SCHIN Ltd)
Bede House, All Saints Business Centre
Newcastle upon Tyne NE1 2ES
Tel: 0191 243 6100
Website: www.cks.library.nhs.uk

A website mainly for GPs giving information for patients listed by disease plus named self-help organisations.

Lung Association
175 Courtwood Crescent, Suite 300
Ottawa, ON K2C 2B5
Canada
Tel: +1 613 569 6411
Website: www.lung.ca

Combats both disease and environmental threats to the lungs. Primary work involves research, education and the promotion of healthy living. A non-profit and volunteer-based organisation.

National Institute for Health and Clinical Excellence (NICE)
MidCity Place, 71 High Holborn
London WC1V 6NA
Tel: 020 7067 5800
Website: www.nice.org.uk

Provides national guidance on the promotion of good health and the prevention and treatment of ill health. Patient information leaflets are available for each piece of guidance issued.

NHS Direct
Tel: 0845 4647 (24 hours, 365 days a year)
Website: www.nhsdirect.nhs.uk

Offers confidential health-care advice, information and referral service. A good first port of call for any health advice.

NHS Smoking Helplines

Freephone: 0800 169 0169
(7am–11pm, 365 days a year)
Pregnancy smoking helpline: 0800 169 9169
(12 noon–9pm, 365 days a year)
Website: www.givingupsmoking.co.uk

Have advice, help and encouragement on giving up smoking. Specialist advisers available to offer on-going support to those who genuinely are trying to give up smoking. Can refer to local branches.

Quit (Smoking Quitlines)

211 Old Street
London EC1V 9NR
Helpline: 0800 002200 (9am–9pm, 365 days a year)
Tel: 020 7251 1551
Website: www.quit.org.uk
Scotland: 0800 848484
Wales: 0800 169 0169 (NHS)

Offers individual advice on giving up smoking in English and Asian languages. Talks to schools on smoking and pregnancy and can refer to local support groups. Runs training courses for professionals.

United States National Library of Medicine

8600 Rockville Pike, Bethesda
MD 20894
USA
Tel: +1 301 594 5983
Website: www.nlm.nih.gov

The world's largest medical library. Collects materials and provides information and research services in all areas of biomedicine and health care.

Websites
BBC
www.bbc.co.uk/health
A helpful website: easy to navigate and offers lots of useful advice and information. Also contains links to other related topics.

Patient UK
www.patient.co.uk
Patient care website.

The internet as a further source of information

After reading this book, you may feel that you would like further information on the subject. The internet is of course an excellent place to look and there are many websites with useful information about medical disorders, related charities and support groups.

For those who do not have a computer at home some bars and cafes offer facilities for accessing the internet. These are listed in the *Yellow Pages* under 'Internet Bars and Cafes' and 'Internet Providers'. Your local library offers a similar facility and has staff to help you find the information that you need.

It should always be remembered, however, that the internet is unregulated and anyone is free to set up a website and add information to it. Many websites offer impartial advice and information that has been compiled and checked by qualified medical professionals. Some, on the other hand, are run by commercial organisations with the purpose of promoting their own products. Others still are run by pressure groups, some of which will provide carefully assessed and accurate information whereas others may be suggesting medications or treatments that are not supported by the medical and scientific community.

Unless you know the address of the website you want to visit – for example, www.familydoctor.co.uk – you may find the following guidelines useful when searching the internet for information.

Search engines and other searchable sites

Google (www.google.co.uk) is the most popular search engine used in the UK, followed by Yahoo! (http://uk.yahoo.com) and MSN (www.msn.co.uk). Also popular are the search engines provided by Internet Service Providers such as Tiscali and other sites such as the BBC site (www.bbc.co.uk).

In addition to the search engines that index the whole web, there are also medical sites with search facilities, which act almost like mini-search engines, but cover only medical topics or even a particular area of medicine. Again, it is wise to look at who is responsible for compiling the information offered to ensure that it is impartial and medically accurate. The NHS Direct site (www.nhsdirect.nhs.uk) is an example of a searchable medical site.

Links to many British medical charities can be found at the Association of Medical Research Charities' website (www.amrc.org.uk) and at Charity Choice (www.charitychoice.co.uk).

Search phrases

Be specific when entering a search phrase. Searching for information on 'cancer' will return results for many different types of cancer as well as on cancer in general. You may even find sites offering astrological information. More useful results will be returned by using search phrases such as 'lung cancer' and 'treatments for lung cancer'. Both Google and Yahoo! offer an advanced search option that includes the ability to search for the exact phrase, enclosing the search phrase in quotes, that is, 'treatments for lung cancer' will have the same effect. Limiting a search to an exact phrase reduces the number of results returned but it is best to refine a search to an exact match only if you are not getting useful results with a normal search. Adding 'UK' to your search term will bring up mainly British sites, so a good phrase might be 'lung cancer' UK (don't include UK within the quotes).

Always remember that the internet is international and unregulated. It holds a wealth of valuable information but individual sites may be biased, out of date or just plain wrong. Family Doctor Publications accepts no responsibility for the content of links published in this series.

Index

Your pages

We have included the following pages because they may help you manage your illness or condition and its treatment.

Before an appointment with a health professional, it can be useful to write down a short list of questions of things that you do not understand, so that you can make sure that you do not forget anything.

Some of the sections may not be relevant to your circumstances.

We are always pleased to receive constructive criticism or suggestions about how to improve the books. You can contact us at:

Email: familydoctor@btinternet.com
Letter: Family Doctor Publications
         PO Box 4664
         Poole
         BH15 1NN

Thank you

Health-care contact details

Name:

Job title:

Place of work:

Tel:

Name:

Job title:

Place of work:

Tel:

Name:

Job title:

Place of work:

Tel:

Name:

Job title:

Place of work:

Tel:

Significant past health events – illnesses/operations/investigations/treatments

Event	Month	Year	Age (at time)

Appointments for health care

Name:

Place:

Date:

Time:

Tel:

Name:

Place:

Date:

Time:

Tel:

Name:

Place:

Date:

Time:

Tel:

Name:

Place:

Date:

Time:

Tel:

Appointments for health care

Name:

Place:

Date:

Time:

Tel:

Name:

Place:

Date:

Time:

Tel:

Name:

Place:

Date:

Time:

Tel:

Name:

Place:

Date:

Time:

Tel:

Current medication(s) prescribed by your doctor

Medicine name:

Purpose:

Frequency & dose:

Start date:

End date:

Medicine name:

Purpose:

Frequency & dose:

Start date:

End date:

Medicine name:

Purpose:

Frequency & dose:

Start date:

End date:

Medicine name:

Purpose:

Frequency & dose:

Start date:

End date:

Other medicines/supplements you are taking, not prescribed by your doctor

Medicine/treatment:

Purpose:

Frequency & dose:

Start date:

End date:

Medicine/treatment:

Purpose:

Frequency & dose:

Start date:

End date:

Medicine/treatment:

Purpose:

Frequency & dose:

Start date:

End date:

Medicine/treatment:

Purpose:

Frequency & dose:

Start date:

End date:

Questions to ask at appointments
(Note: do bear in mind that doctors work under great time pressure, so long lists may not be helpful for either of you)

Questions to ask at appointments
(Note: do bear in mind that doctors work under great time pressure, so long lists may not be helpful for either of you)

Notes